THE COMPLETE LOW BACK PAIN SOLUTION

EVIDENCE-BASED GUIDE TO RELIEF AND LONG-TERM RECOVERY THROUGH TARGETED EXERCISES AND LIFESTYLE CHANGES

DR. K.D. CHRISTENSEN

CONTENTS

INTRODUCTION

As a retired Sports Chiropractor with over four decades of experience, I've witnessed countless patients struggle with debilitating lower back pain. One particular case stands out in my memory—a young athlete, once full of promise, now sidelined by chronic pain. It was a turning point in my career, a moment that crystallized the need for a comprehensive, evidence-based guide to help people like her find lasting relief.

I'm Dr. K.D. Christensen, and throughout my 40-year journey in chiropractic care and rehabilitation, including a decade working in a hospital setting, I've seen firsthand the impact that targeted interventions and lifestyle changes can have on lower back pain. This book represents the culmination of my expertise, passion, and dedication to helping others reclaim their lives from the grip of chronic pain.

"The Complete Low Back Pain Solution" is more than just another self-help book; it's an evidence-based roadmap to relief and long-term recovery. By integrating the latest scientific research with practical, actionable strategies, this guide offers a holistic approach to managing and preventing lower back pain. Whether you're an adult, athlete, or youth, the targeted exercises and lifestyle modifications detailed within these pages can be tailored to your unique needs and fitness level.

Inside, you'll find a wealth of information and tools, including:

- Detailed exercise programs designed to strengthen, stabilize, and mobilize the spine
- Lifestyle modifications to reduce pain and prevent future flare-ups
- Success stories from real people who have overcome lower back pain
- Strategies for cultivating mental resilience and emotional well-being

By emphasizing an evidence-based approach, "The Complete Low Back Pain Solution" sets itself apart from the myriad of unsubstantiated quick fixes and miracle cures that often leave sufferers frustrated and searching for real solutions. The methods and techniques outlined in this book are grounded in scientific studies and clinical experience, ensuring that you're equipped with reliable, effective strategies for managing your pain.

My motivation for writing this book stems from a deep-seated desire to empower others to take control of their back health. Having witnessed the transformative power of education and self-management, I firmly believe that with the right tools and knowledge, anyone can achieve pain-free living. It's my sincere hope that by sharing my expertise and insights, I can guide you on your journey to improved spine health and overall well-being.

As you delve into the pages of this book, I encourage you to approach the content with an open mind and a commitment to action. The path to recovery requires dedication and consistency, but the rewards—a life unburdened by chronic pain—are well worth the effort. By actively engaging with the exercises, lifestyle modifications, and mental strategies presented, you'll be taking a proactive step towards reclaiming your health and vitality.

So, whether you're seeking relief from a recent injury or looking to break free from the cycle of chronic pain, "The Complete Low Back Pain Solution" is your comprehensive guide to a stronger, healthier spine. With the perfect blend of scientific evidence, practical advice, and inspirational stories, this book will be your trusted companion on the road to recovery. Let's embark on this transformative journey together, one page at a time.

1

UNDERSTANDING YOUR BACK PAIN

There's a moment in life when the reality of persistent back pain hits home—a moment when simple acts like tying shoelaces or lifting a grocery bag feel like monumental tasks. It was during such an encounter with a patient, struggling with the limitations imposed by relentless back pain, that I fully appreciated the complexity and the often-overlooked intricacies of the human spine. This encounter fueled my determination to create a guide that not only addresses the symptoms but dives into the depths of understanding the very structure that supports us throughout our lives. By comprehending the anatomy of your lower back, you gain the power to reclaim your body and your life. Let's explore how these structures work and what happens when they don't.

1.1 ANATOMY OF THE LOWER BACK: A USER-FRIENDLY GUIDE

The lower back, or lumbar region, serves as the foundation of our body's architecture. Comprised of five vertebrae, labeled L1 to L5, this section of the spine bears the weight of the upper body, providing both stability and mobility. These vertebrae are robust, each stacked upon the next, forming a gentle inward curve known as the lordotic curve, which contributes to balance and shock absorption. Nestled between these vertebrae are intervertebral discs, acting as cushion-like shock absorbers that allow for flexibility and movement. These discs are pivotal, yet they are also prone to wear and tear, sometimes leading to conditions such as herniated discs. The spinal cord, a delicate bundle of nerves encased within these protective vertebrae, extends down to the first lumbar vertebra, after which the cauda equina, a collection of nerve roots, continues to innervate the lower body. These nerves play a crucial role in controlling leg movement and transmitting sensory information from the lower extremities.

Beyond the bony structure, a network of muscles and ligaments lends additional support and movement capabilities to the spine. The erector spinae muscles, running alongside the vertebral column, are essential for maintaining posture and allowing for bending and twisting motions. These powerful muscles work tirelessly to keep us upright and must be strong and flexible to prevent strain.

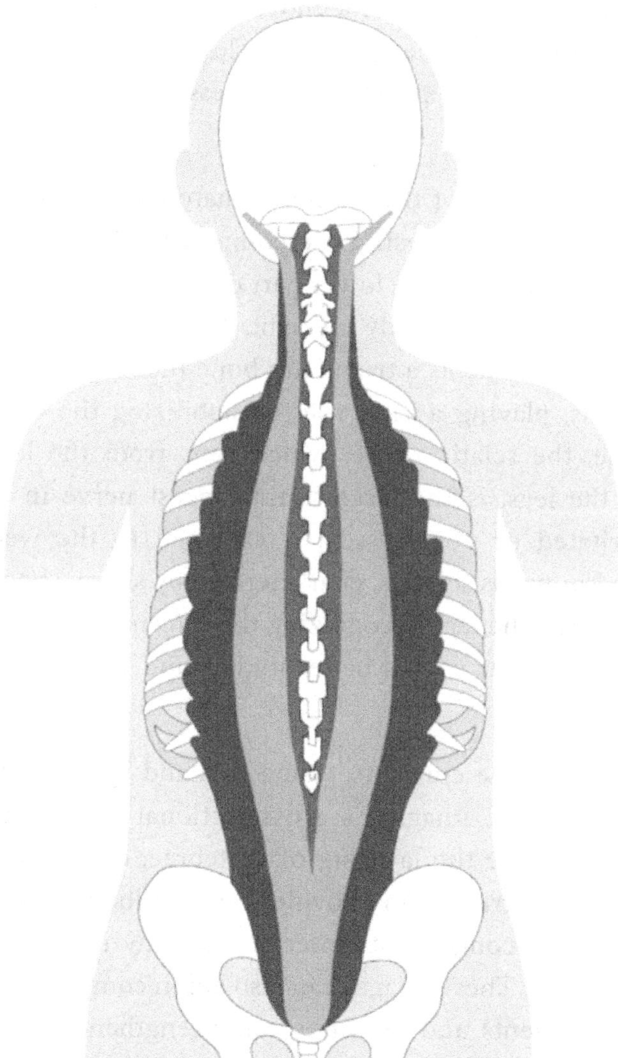

Fig 1.1 Erector Spinae Muscles

Similarly, the ligamentum flavum, a band of elastic tissue connecting the vertebrae, plays an integral role in maintaining spinal stability during motion. Other ligaments, such as the anterior and posterior longitudinal ligaments, add another layer of stability, ensuring the vertebrae move synchronously and without slipping out of place. When these muscles and ligaments are functioning optimally, they provide the necessary support to prevent injury and pain.

Understanding some of the common anatomical terms related to the lower back can demystify the complexity of this region. The lumbar region refers to the lower part of the spine, responsible for supporting most of the body's weight. The sacrum, located below the lumbar vertebrae, is a triangular bone that connects the spine to the pelvis, playing a vital role in stabilizing the upper body. Meanwhile, the sciatic nerve, which runs from the lower back down to the legs, is the largest and longest nerve in the body. When irritated or compressed, it can lead to the well-known condition known as sciatica, characterized by sharp, shooting pain radiating down the leg. Recognizing these terms and their significance can empower you to better understand your diagnosis and treatment options.

To fully grasp these concepts, visual aids and illustrations can be immensely helpful. Imagine a cross-sectional view of the spine, where you can see the layering of vertebrae, discs, muscles, and nerves. Such diagrams can provide clarity, allowing you to visualize how these components interact and why maintaining their health is crucial. These images can also aid in comprehending how certain movements and exercises can strengthen or strain these structures, providing a clearer picture of the path to recovery and prevention. By familiarizing yourself with the anatomy of your lower back, you take the first step towards a more in-depth understanding of the root causes of your pain and the effective strategies to combat it.

1.2 COMMON CAUSES OF LOWER BACK PAIN ACROSS AGE GROUPS

Lower back pain, an ailment that knows no age boundaries, manifests differently as we progress through life's stages. In youth, growth spurts and sports injuries are prevalent culprits. During these rapid phases of growth, the body sometimes struggles to keep up with the demands placed upon it. Young athletes, eager to excel, often push their bodies beyond their limits, leading to strains and sprains. Picture a high school gymnast practicing her routine: a slight miscalculation in a flip can mean weeks of recovery. These injuries not only disrupt their athletic ambitions but also their daily lives, affecting school and social activities. The importance of teaching proper techniques and encouraging rest becomes paramount in reducing these incidents.

For adults, particularly those in the workforce, occupational hazards become the primary source of discomfort. The modern office environment, with its ergonomic challenges, often contributes to back pain. Many of us are guilty of slouching over computers or using poorly adjusted chairs, unaware of the toll this takes on our spines. Similarly, those in physically demanding jobs may not utilize proper lifting techniques, leading to cumulative strain. Imagine a warehouse worker who routinely lifts heavy boxes without bending at the knees; each lift adds stress, eventually resulting in significant pain. Educating individuals on ergonomic setups and safe lifting practices can mitigate these risks, fostering a healthier work environment.

As we age, degenerative conditions become more prominent, with seniors facing the wear and tear of a lifetime. Conditions such as arthritis and spinal stenosis often surface, and the aging body's reduced ability to repair itself exacerbates these issues. For many seniors, simple activities like gardening or walking can become arduous tasks. The gradual decline in bone density and joint flexibility requires attention and care, emphasizing the need for gentle, regular exercise to maintain mobility and reduce pain. Understanding these age-specific causes allows us to tailor interventions that are both effective and compassionate, recognizing the unique challenges faced at each stage of life.

Across all age groups, posture and ergonomics play a critical role in maintaining spine health. Poor posture, often developed from prolonged sitting or incorrect standing, places undue strain on the lumbar region. A desk job may seem harmless, but without proper chair support and desk height, workers find themselves with chronic back pain. Similarly, improper ergonomics at home, like slouching on a couch, contributes to discomfort. Teaching individuals to adjust their environments—raising a computer monitor to eye level or using lumbar supports—can significantly alleviate these issues. Simple changes, though seemingly minor, can have profound impacts on long-term health.

Physical activity, while beneficial in many respects, can also be a double-edged sword when not executed correctly. Maintaining an active lifestyle is crucial for overall well-being, yet improper exercise techniques can lead to injuries. Overuse injuries are common among those who exercise without adequate rest or variation in their routines. Consider the weekend warrior who jumps into intense workouts after a sedentary week; without proper warm-up or technique, they become susceptible to muscle strains. It's vital to educate on the importance of form and balance, encouraging activities that strengthen and stretch the back without overexerting it.

Environmental and lifestyle factors further compound the likelihood of developing lower back pain. A sedentary lifestyle, marked by long hours of inactivity, weakens the muscles that support the spine. Meanwhile, poor mattress quality affects sleep posture, leading to morning stiffness and discomfort. Imagine waking up each day with a sore back, a direct result of inadequate support during sleep. Encouraging a shift towards more active lifestyles and investing in quality sleep surfaces can reduce the prevalence of these pain sources. Awareness and proactive adjustments in daily habits can significantly improve back health, offering relief and prevention.

1.3 THE SCIENCE OF SPINE HEALTH: WHY IT MATTERS

The spine serves as the body's central scaffold, supporting weight, enabling movement, and protecting the spinal cord. Its intricate design allows us to perform an array of activities, from simple tasks like getting out of bed to more complex movements like running or jumping. The spine's load-bearing capacity is nothing short of remarkable. It balances the demands of strength and flexibility, absorbing shocks and distributing forces evenly across its length. Imagine it as a suspension bridge, where each vertebra acts like a cable, bearing the tension and weight of the entire structure. This analogy helps us appreciate the spine's ability to withstand the pressures of daily life, but it also underscores the importance of maintaining its integrity. A well-functioning spine supports our physical activities and contributes significantly to overall health.

Proper spinal alignment is crucial for optimal function. When the spine maintains its natural curves, it operates efficiently, minimizing strain on muscles and ligaments. This alignment ensures that the vertebrae and discs remain in place, offering a stable base for movement. In contrast, misalignment can lead to a cascade of issues. It can compress nerves, leading to pain and discomfort, and can even affect other systems in the body. The concept of a neutral spine position—where the spine's natural curves are preserved—

becomes paramount in avoiding these complications. By promoting good posture and alignment, we can prevent many of the common problems associated with back pain. These practices are not just about standing tall, but about maintaining the health of the nervous system and ensuring efficient communication between the brain and body.

Recent scientific studies have shed light on effective interventions for spine health. Research on core strengthening has shown that a strong core supports the spine, reducing the risk of injury and pain. A robust core acts like a natural brace, stabilizing the spine during movement. Moreover, studies on stretching highlight its role in maintaining flexibility, reducing muscle tension, and preventing injury. Stretching keeps the muscles around the spine supple, allowing for greater range of motion without strain. These evidence-based strategies offer practical solutions for enhancing spine health and alleviating pain. By incorporating these findings into daily routines, we can make significant strides in preventing and managing back pain.

The spine's influence extends beyond the musculoskeletal system. Its health impacts the nervous system, which relies on an unobstructed spinal column to transmit signals throughout the body. Nerve compression or irritation due to spine issues can lead to pain, numbness, and weakness. The spine also plays a role in cardiovascular health. Studies have found that poor posture and spinal alignment can affect circulation and respiratory function, emphasizing the need for comprehensive spine care. Maintaining a healthy spine, therefore, supports overall physiological function, affecting everything from energy levels to stress management. By prioritizing spine health, we address pain and enhance our well-being, opening doors to a more active and fulfilling life.

1.4 IDENTIFYING YOUR PAIN: SELF-ASSESSMENT TOOLS

Understanding your back pain begins with the ability to assess it accurately. Self-assessment tools are invaluable in this process, providing you with a clearer picture of what's happening in your body. One practical tool is a pain diary, a simple yet effective way to track your pain over time. In a small notebook or even a digital app, jot down the times when pain occurs, its intensity, and any activities that may have triggered it. Over days or weeks, patterns will emerge, offering insights into your pain's behavior. This diary aids you in pinpointing potential causes and serves as a valuable resource when consulting healthcare professionals. The goal is to identify triggers and recognize patterns, transforming vague sensations into specific data that can guide your path to recovery.

Interpreting pain signals is another crucial aspect of managing your condition effectively. Pain can manifest in various forms, each telling a different story about what's happening within. Sharp pain might signify a sudden injury or strain, something that requires immediate attention. In contrast, dull pain often indicates ongoing issues, perhaps related to posture or repetitive stress. Radiating pain, which travels from one area to another, could suggest nerve involvement, such as with sciatica. Localized pain, confined to a specific region, might point to muscle tension or a joint problem. Recognizing these distinctions empowers you to respond appropriately, whether by adjusting your daily activities or seeking professional advice. It's about listening to your body and understanding its language.

To facilitate early intervention, a preliminary diagnosis checklist can be immensely helpful. This checklist encourages you to note the frequency and duration of pain episodes. Is the pain constant, or does it come and go? Does it intensify after certain activities or at specific times of the day? Identifying what relieves your pain—such as rest, heat, or gentle stretching—can also offer clues about its nature. This information is crucial. It helps you and your healthcare provider determine the best course of action, whether that involves lifestyle adjustments, exercises, or further medical evaluation. By systematically gathering this data, you arm yourself with the knowledge needed to make informed decisions about your health.

While self-assessment is a powerful tool, it's important to remember the role of professional diagnosis. Self-evaluation can sometimes lead to misinterpretations or overlook serious issues. For instance, persistent pain that doesn't improve with home remedies or exhibits unusual characteristics, such as numbness or weakness, warrants professional attention. Consulting with a healthcare provider ensures that underlying conditions are identified and addressed appropriately. They can perform thorough assessments, using advanced diagnostic tools to pinpoint the exact cause of your pain. This step is crucial in preventing further injury and ensuring that you receive the most effective treatment. So, when should you seek medical advice? If you experience severe pain, symptoms that persist despite self-care, or any signs of nerve involvement like tingling or weakness, it's time to consult a professional. They can provide the clarity and guidance needed to navigate your path to recovery.

Recognizing the nuances of your pain through self-assessment empowers you to take charge of your health. By employing these tools—pain diaries, interpretative skills, and checklists—you create a foundation for understanding your condition. This proactive approach aids in managing your current pain and in preventing future episodes. It's about becoming attuned to your body's signals and taking informed steps towards relief and recovery.

1.5 CHRONIC VS. ACUTE PAIN: UNDERSTANDING THE DIFFERENCE

Pain is a universal experience, yet its nuances can be as varied as the individuals who endure it. Two primary classifications—chronic and acute pain—help us delineate these experiences, providing clarity on their nature and management. Acute pain, transient and sudden, often acts as the body's alarm system. It signals injury or a potential threat, urging immediate attention. This type of pain typically lasts less than three months and diminishes as the underlying cause heals. Consider the sharp sting of a muscle strain after an intense workout, or the throbbing ache from a minor back injury. These examples of acute pain are typically linked to identifiable events or actions, such as lifting a heavy object improperly, and they often resolve with rest and simple interventions.

Conversely, chronic pain lingers, persisting beyond the typical healing time, often extending for months or even years. It can stem from an initial injury, like a herniated disc, or manifest without a clear cause, becoming a condition in itself. Chronic pain is relentless, often varying in intensity but rarely disappearing entirely. This persistence can wear down even the most resilient individuals, making daily tasks burdensome. The ongoing nature of chronic pain necessitates a different approach, focusing on long-term management rather than quick fixes. Understanding these distinctions is crucial in setting realistic expectations and crafting effective treatment plans.

The implications of differentiating between acute and chronic pain are significant. For acute pain, immediate relief is often the goal. Treatments might include rest, ice or heat applications, and over-the-counter pain relief. These strategies aim to address the immediate discomfort and promote healing. In contrast, managing chronic pain requires a more holistic approach. It involves a combination of therapies, such as physical therapy, medications, lifestyle changes, and sometimes psychological support. Chronic pain often benefits from a personalized plan, tailored to the individual's specific needs and circumstances, focusing on improving function and quality of life rather than complete elimination of pain.

Chronic pain also presents unique psychological challenges. The constant presence of pain can lead to feelings of frustration, anxiety, and even depression. These mental health concerns can exacerbate the perception of pain, creating a vicious cycle that can be difficult to break. Addressing these psychological aspects is as important as treating the physical symptoms. Cognitive-behavioral therapy and other forms of psychological support can provide individuals with coping mechanisms, helping them manage not only their pain, but also the emotional toll it exacts. Acknowledging the mental health challenges associated with chronic pain is a vital step in comprehensive care.

Examples of conditions often classified under these pain types further illustrate their differences. Acute pain might arise from a muscle strain, where the pain is immediate and linked to a specific incident. A herniated disc, however, can lead to chronic pain, with persistent discomfort that might radiate into the legs, affecting mobility and daily activities. These conditions highlight the need for targeted interventions. While acute pain might resolve with time and conservative measures, chronic pain often requires ongoing management to mitigate its impact on life. Understanding these categories clarifies the path forward, guiding individuals and healthcare providers in choosing the most appropriate strategies to manage pain effectively. Through this knowledge, a clearer path to relief and improved quality of life emerges.

1.6 THE ROLE OF LIFESTYLE IN BACK PAIN DEVELOPMENT

In the hustle of daily life, we often overlook how our routine habits shape our physical well-being. Yet, these seemingly innocuous activities can have profound effects on our backs. Consider the hours spent hunched over a desk, absorbed in work, oblivious to posture. This common scenario exemplifies how poor sitting habits insidiously contribute to back discomfort. A chair lacking proper lumbar support or a monitor positioned too low can cause the spine to curve unnaturally, leading to strain and eventual pain. Similarly, footwear choices bear scrutiny. Shoes lacking adequate support or cushioning force the spine to compensate for imbalance, transferring stress to the lower back. Elegant yet unsupportive footwear, often favored for style over comfort, can exacerbate these issues, highlighting the need for thoughtful choices in daily attire.

Diet and nutrition play pivotal roles beyond their obvious health benefits, directly influencing inflammation and muscle integrity. Certain foods, rich in antioxidants and omega-3 fatty acids, combat inflammation, a common contributor to back pain. Incorporating anti-inflammatory foods such as leafy greens, nuts, and fatty fish can mitigate these effects, promoting a healthier spine. Additionally, calcium and vitamin D intake are crucial for maintaining bone strength. These nutrients support vertebral health, preventing degenerative conditions that may lead to pain. A diet rich in these elements not only fosters overall health but also safeguards against back-related ailments, underscoring the interconnectedness of nutrition and spinal health.

Sleep is another cornerstone of back health, yet its significance is often underestimated. The position one adopts during slumber can either support or strain the spine. A mattress that's too firm or too soft fails to maintain the spine's natural alignment, resulting in stiffness and discomfort upon waking. Selecting a mattress that supports the body's contours, coupled with a sleep position that aligns the spine, can alleviate such issues. Equally important is addressing stress, which often exacerbates physical pain. Stress prompts muscle tension, particularly in the back, increasing discomfort. Simple stress-reduction techniques—deep breathing, meditation, or even a short daily walk—can significantly ease this tension, promoting both mental and physical relaxation.

Lifestyle modification doesn't require drastic overhauls. Instead, gradual changes can yield substantial improvements in spine health. Establishing a balanced exercise routine that incorporates strength training, flexibility exercises, and cardiovascular activity fosters a resilient body. Such routines enhance muscle support around the spine, reducing susceptibility to injury. Incorporating mindfulness practices, such as yoga or tai chi, further enhances these benefits, promoting mental clarity and physical balance. These practices encourage body awareness, helping individuals recognize and correct poor habits before they manifest as pain.

The journey to improved back health isn't about perfection; it's about awareness and incremental progress. By evaluating daily habits, making informed choices, and embracing gradual change, you create a foundation for a healthier spine. This proactive approach not only alleviates current discomfort but also fortifies against future challenges. Through mindful living, you unlock the potential for a vibrant, pain-free existence, where your body supports your aspirations, unencumbered by the weight of habitual neglect.

2

LIFESTYLE CHANGES FOR LONG-TERM HEALTH

Picture this: you're at your desk, eyes fixed on your computer screen, shoulders hunched, and back slightly arched. Hours pass without much movement, and by the end of the day, a familiar tightness creeps into your lower back. This scenario is all too common in our modern world, where the demands of work and study often tether us to our desks. Yet, this doesn't have to be the norm. By integrating ergonomic principles into your daily routine, both at home and work, you can transform your environment into a supportive ally for your spine. Ergonomics is not just about comfort; it's about creating a workspace that promotes health and prevents the strain that contributes to back pain.

Ergonomic setups begin with the chair you choose. An ergonomic chair is not merely a seat; it's a foundation for good posture. These chairs are designed to support the natural curve of your spine, encouraging an upright, relaxed position. Look for ones with adjustable height, backrest, and armrests, allowing you to tailor it to your unique needs. The benefits are substantial: reduced pressure on your lower back, improved circulation, and less muscle fatigue throughout the day. Beyond the chair, consider the height of your desk. An improperly adjusted desk can lead to awkward postures, such as slouching or craning your neck. Adjust the desk height so your elbows rest comfortably at a 90-degree angle when typing, keeping your wrists straight and relaxed.

Setting up your workspace doesn't stop there. Monitor placement is crucial. Position your screen at eye level, about an arm's length away. This setup minimizes neck strain and reduces the temptation to hunch forward. Similarly, your keyboard and mouse should be within easy reach, close enough to avoid overextending your arms. Arrange them so your hands are parallel to your forearms, maintaining a neutral wrist position. These adjustments create a seamless workflow, minimizing discomfort and promoting productivity.

Incorporating ergonomic tools and accessories further enhances your setup. A footrest can be particularly beneficial if your feet dangle when seated, providing support and encouraging proper leg alignment. Ergonomic desk mats can also be useful, offering a cushioned surface that reduces pressure on your feet and promotes comfort during long periods of standing. These simple additions can make a significant difference in your daily comfort and spine health.

Ergonomics isn't confined to the office. Apply these principles on the go to maintain spine health wherever you are. For frequent travelers, consider portable lumbar support pillows. These lightweight, inflatable cushions provide much-needed support during car rides or flights, preventing slouching and reducing back strain. When driving, adjust your seat to maintain a slight bend in your knees, and keep the steering wheel within easy reach to avoid leaning forward. These small adjustments ensure that even when you're away from your usual setup, your back remains supported.

Ergonomics is about making thoughtful choices that prioritize your spine's well-being. By being mindful of your posture and environment, you create a supportive atmosphere that alleviates strain and promotes comfort. Take a moment to evaluate your current setup. Are there areas where you could make improvements? Start with one change, such as adjusting your chair or raising your monitor, and observe the difference it makes. Over time, these adjustments become natural, leading to a healthier, more comfortable life, free from the constraints of back pain.

Ergonomic Checklist for Your Workspace

- **Chair**: Adjustable height, backrest, and armrests to support natural spine curvature.
- **Desk**: Set at a height where elbows rest at a 90-degree angle.
- **Monitor**: Positioned at eye level, about an arm's length away.
- **Keyboard and Mouse**: Within easy reach, hands parallel to forearms.
- **Footrest and Desk Mats**: Consider these for added comfort and support.
- **Travel Adjustments**: Use lumbar support in vehicles and adjust car seats for optimal alignment.

2.1 ANTI-INFLAMMATORY DIET: FOODS FOR SPINE HEALTH

Imagine the power of your plate in shaping your spine's health. It's not just about what you eat; it's about how certain foods can act as allies in the battle against inflammation, a common culprit behind chronic pain. Omega-3 fatty acids, found abundantly in salmon and mackerel, are renowned for their anti-inflammatory properties. These healthy fats reduce inflammation, which can alleviate the discomfort associated with back pain. By incorporating fish into your diet a couple of times a week, you're not just enjoying a delicious meal; you're actively supporting your spine's well-being. Equally potent are the antioxidants found in berries. Blueberries, strawberries, and raspberries are not only tasty but also rich in compounds that combat oxidative stress, another factor linked to inflammation. These small fruits pack a mighty punch, helping to keep your body's inflammatory responses in check.

Expanding your diet to include various anti-inflammatory foods can further bolster your efforts. Leafy greens like spinach and kale are nutritional powerhouses, offering a combination of vitamins, minerals, and antioxidants. They're easy to incorporate into meals, whether as a salad base or a cooked side dish. Nuts, such as almonds and walnuts, offer healthy fats and fiber, making them a satisfying snack that supports your spine. These foods, with their myriad of benefits, should become staples in your kitchen. They support spinal health and contribute to overall wellness, offering protection against a range of ailments.

When planning meals, focusing on anti-inflammatory ingredients can make all the difference. Batch cooking is a practical approach, saving time while ensuring you have healthy options readily available. Consider preparing a large pot of vegetable stew, rich with anti-inflammatory spices like turmeric and ginger, which add flavor and enhance your body's ability to fight inflammation. Smoothies offer another convenient way to incorporate these foods into your diet. Blend together berries, leafy greens, and a splash of almond milk for a nutrient-packed drink that you can enjoy on the go. These strategies make it easier to maintain an anti-inflammatory diet, even with a busy lifestyle.

Supplements can also play a role in managing inflammation, though they should complement, not replace, a healthy diet. Turmeric capsules, with the active ingredient curcumin, are popular for their anti-inflammatory effects. Similarly, fish oil supplements provide a concentrated source of omega-3 fatty acids. However, it's important to consult a healthcare provider before introducing new supplements into your routine. They can offer guidance on appropriate dosages and ensure there are no interactions with other medications you might be taking. This personalized advice helps you make informed choices that align with your health goals.

With each meal, you have the opportunity to support your spine's health. By choosing foods that fight inflammation, you take an active role in preventing and managing back pain. Nutrition is a powerful tool, one that complements other lifestyle changes in your journey towards a healthier back. Enjoying a colorful, varied diet satisfies your taste buds and fortifies your body, laying the foundation for long-term spine health.

2.2 DAILY HABITS THAT PREVENT BACK PAIN

In today's fast-paced world, it's easy to overlook the small habits that can make a big difference in your spinal health. One of the simplest yet most effective strategies is to incorporate regular standing breaks throughout your day. Whether you're working at a desk, studying, or binge-watching your favorite series, standing up every 30 minutes can help alleviate the buildup of pressure in your lower back. This brief pause allows your muscles to stretch and your spine to decompress, reducing the risk of stiffness and pain. Conscious posture checks are equally important. By taking a moment to adjust your posture—whether sitting or standing—you can ensure your spine maintains its natural curves, preventing unnecessary strain. This practice becomes second nature with consistency, promoting a healthier back over time.

Movement is another vital component in maintaining a healthy spine. Integrating physical activity into your daily routine doesn't require a complete overhaul of your schedule. Simple changes, like opting for walking meetings instead of sitting down or choosing to stand during phone calls, can make a significant difference. These activities encourage dynamic movement, which helps strengthen your back and core muscles while improving circulation. Even small stretches during TV commercials or while waiting for your coffee to brew can add up, providing your spine with the flexibility and strength it needs to support your body effectively. The goal is to create a rhythm of movement that complements your lifestyle, making it easier to stay active without feeling overwhelmed.

Stress management is crucial not only for mental well-being but also for maintaining a pain-free back. Stress often manifests physically, leading to muscle tension and exacerbating back pain. Implementing quick stress relief techniques, such as deep breathing exercises, can help you manage these stress-induced tensions. Simple practices like inhaling deeply through your nose, holding for a few seconds, and exhaling slowly can calm your nervous system and relax your muscles. Incorporating mindfulness practices, such as meditation or yoga, further enhances this effect, providing a holistic approach to stress reduction. These practices don't require a significant time investment but offer substantial benefits, allowing you to face daily challenges with a clearer mind and more relaxed body.

A balanced lifestyle is about more than just physical activity and stress management; it's an integration of physical, mental, and emotional health. Setting realistic daily goals can help structure your day, providing a sense of accomplishment and purpose without overwhelming you. These goals could be as simple as taking a 5-minute walk every hour or dedicating 10 minutes to meditation before bed. Prioritizing self-care is equally important. This doesn't mean indulging in luxury but rather finding moments to nurture yourself, whether through a hobby, reading, or simply relaxing. By combining these elements, you create a supportive environment for your spine and overall well-being. Each small step you take contributes to a healthier, more balanced lifestyle.

The cumulative effect of these daily habits is profound. By making conscious choices to move more, manage stress effectively, and balance your lifestyle, you provide your spine with the support it needs to remain strong and healthy. These practices don't require drastic changes but rather a mindful approach to your everyday activities. Over time, they become ingrained in your routine, leading to a life with less pain and greater mobility.

2.3 DECOMPRESSING YOUR SPINE: TECHNIQUES FOR DAILY RELIEF

Imagine your spine as a tightly wound spring, carrying the weight of your daily activities. Over time, pressure builds, leading to discomfort and pain. Spinal decompression offers a way to alleviate this pressure, providing relief by gently elongating the spine. This process enhances the space between your vertebrae, reducing pressure on discs and nerves. As pressure diminishes, circulation improves, delivering nutrients and oxygen to spinal tissues. This increased blood flow fosters healing and reduces stiffness, offering a respite from the discomfort that often accompanies a long day.

Incorporating simple decompression exercises into your routine can be transformative. One effective method is hanging from a pull-up bar. This exercise uses gravity to naturally stretch the spine, allowing it to decompress. Simply grip the bar, letting your body hang freely. Your feet should be off the ground, with arms fully extended. Hold this position for twenty to thirty seconds, feeling the gentle pull as your spine lengthens. Alternatively, an inversion table can aid decompression. By securely attaching your feet and inverting your body, gravity assists in stretching the spine. This technique alleviates disc pressure and enhances overall flexibility. As you incorporate these exercises, you'll notice a marked improvement in your spine's resilience and comfort.

To make decompression a staple of your daily routine, consider integrating short breaks throughout your day. These breaks allow you to step away from your tasks, engage in a quick stretch, and let gravity do its work. You might find that a few minutes of hanging from a bar during a lunch break or a brief session on an inversion table in the evening can significantly ease tension. By making these practices a regular part of your day, you fortify your spine against the cumulative stress of daily life. Over time, these moments of decompression become second nature, seamlessly blending into your daily rhythm.

For some, professional decompression therapies offer additional support. Chiropractic spinal adjustments, for instance, can realign the vertebrae, further reducing pressure on nerves and improving mobility. These adjustments, performed by trained professionals, provide targeted relief, addressing specific areas of tension and imbalance. Physical therapy sessions also offer tailored decompression strategies, combining exercises and manual techniques to enhance spine health. A physical therapist can assess your unique needs, crafting a personalized approach to decompression that complements your lifestyle. These professional interventions can be particularly beneficial if at-home exercises don't fully address your discomfort, offering you a comprehensive strategy for maintaining a healthy spine.

2.4 SLEEP AND SPINE HEALTH: FINDING THE PERFECT POSITION

The way you sleep profoundly influences your spine's health. Sleep quality and your sleeping position are critical in determining how well your spine recovers from the day's activities. When you sleep, your body enters a state of repair and regeneration, making it a prime time for addressing spinal issues. Proper spinal alignment during rest is crucial because it ensures that no part of your spine is under undue stress. Misalignment can exacerbate pain and hinder recovery, leading to a cycle of discomfort that persists day after day. The position you choose can either alleviate this stress or compound it, making it essential to find a posture that supports your spine's natural curves.

Side sleeping is often recommended for its benefits to spinal alignment. By placing a pillow between your knees, you help maintain a neutral spine position, preventing the top leg from pulling the spine out of alignment. This simple adjustment can reduce pressure on the lower back and hips, promoting a more restful sleep. For those who prefer sleeping on their back, placing a pillow under your knees can achieve a similar effect. This position supports the natural curve of the lower back, distributing weight evenly and minimizing strain. It's about finding what feels comfortable while also supporting your spine's needs.

Choosing the right mattress and pillow can make all the difference in achieving a good night's sleep. A medium-firm mattress usually provides the best support, balancing comfort and spine alignment. It should be firm enough to support the natural curves of the spine but soft enough to relieve pressure points. Contoured pillows can also play a significant role in maintaining proper neck and upper spine alignment. These pillows curve around your neck, offering targeted support that helps prevent strain. Investing in quality bedding tailored to your sleeping preferences ensures that your spine receives the support it requires throughout the night.

Improving sleep quality goes beyond just physical adjustments; it's also about creating a conducive environment for rest. Establishing a bedtime routine can signal your body that it's time to unwind, making it easier to fall asleep and stay asleep. This could include activities like reading a book, taking a warm bath, or practicing relaxation techniques. Reducing screen time before bed is another effective strategy. The blue light emitted by phones and tablets can disrupt your body's natural sleep-wake cycle, making it harder to fall asleep. By turning off devices at least an hour before bedtime, you help your body transition smoothly into a restful state.

2.5 HYDRATION AND MUSCLE FUNCTION: STAYING FLUID

Water is the lifeblood of our muscles. Imagine every movement you make—whether it's reaching for a book or sprinting down a track—powered by the almost magical interplay of muscles and water. Staying hydrated ensures your muscles remain elastic and responsive, crucial for preventing cramps and strains. When your body is well-hydrated, your muscles can contract and relax efficiently, reducing the risk of fatigue and injury. Think of water as the lubricant that keeps your muscular engine running smoothly. Without it, muscles become stiff, and their ability to support the spine diminishes, potentially leading to discomfort and even injury.

The question then becomes: how much water do you need each day? A simple guideline is to drink eight 8-ounce glasses, which translates to about two liters or half a gallon. However, individual needs can vary based on activity level, climate, and overall health. An easy way to monitor your hydration status is by observing the color of your urine. A pale, straw-like hue typically indicates adequate hydration, whereas darker shades might suggest you need more fluids. This visual cue is a quick and effective method to ensure you're meeting your body's needs. By consistently hydrating, you lay a foundation for overall wellness and spine health.

Incorporating hydration into your daily routine doesn't have to be a chore. Start by keeping a reusable water bottle by your side throughout the day. This constant reminder makes it easy to take sips regularly, preventing dehydration before it starts. Setting reminders on your phone or using a hydration app can also reinforce the habit, ensuring you maintain fluid intake even during busy days. These small adjustments can become second nature, seamlessly integrating into your lifestyle and supporting your spine's health with minimal effort. The goal is not just to drink water, but to make it a habitual part of your day.

Dehydration's impact on back health can be significant. When your body lacks fluids, muscles lose elasticity, becoming more prone to stiffness and reduced flexibility. This rigidity can lead to discomfort, as tight muscles struggle to support the spine adequately. Moreover, dehydration affects the intervertebral discs, which rely on fluid to maintain their height and cushioning ability. Without sufficient hydration, these discs can shrink, leading to increased friction and the potential for degeneration. Over time, this can exacerbate existing back issues or even trigger new ones, emphasizing the importance of regular fluid intake for spinal health. Keeping your body hydrated is a proactive step in maintaining a healthy back.

As you consider the role of hydration in your daily life, remember that it's not just about quenching thirst. It's about supporting every system in your body, from muscles to nerves, ensuring they function optimally. By prioritizing hydration, you take a vital step in safeguarding your spine and overall health. Water is more than just a beverage; it's an essential partner in your quest for a pain-free life.

3

EVIDENCE-BASED EXERCISE PROGRAMS

Imagine the thrill of crossing the finish line, the crowd's energy echoing around you. For athletes, each moment is not just about the win, but about the rigorous preparation that makes it possible. Yet, with the glory of athleticism comes the constant dance between peak performance and injury prevention. It's this delicate balance that forms the core of athlete-specific recovery exercises—an approach that acknowledges the unique demands sports place on the body.

Athletes juggle the need to maintain high performance with the necessity of recovery. This balance is paramount; training too hard without adequate recovery can lead to overuse injuries, while insufficient training might miss the mark of peak performance. Recovery isn't merely about rest. It's an active process involving exercises that enhance flexibility and aid muscle recovery. Flexibility is not a luxury; it's a necessity that allows athletes to push boundaries safely. By incorporating regular stretching into your routine, you ensure muscles remain supple and responsive.

Stretching primes your muscles for performance, reducing the risk of strains and enhancing efficiency.

Identifying key muscle groups and targeting them with specific exercises is crucial for athletes. The hamstrings and hip flexors are often under significant stress in sports like running, soccer, and cycling. These muscles are involved in almost every movement an athlete makes, from sprinting to squatting. Regular hamstring stretches ensure these muscles remain flexible, reducing the risk of strains.

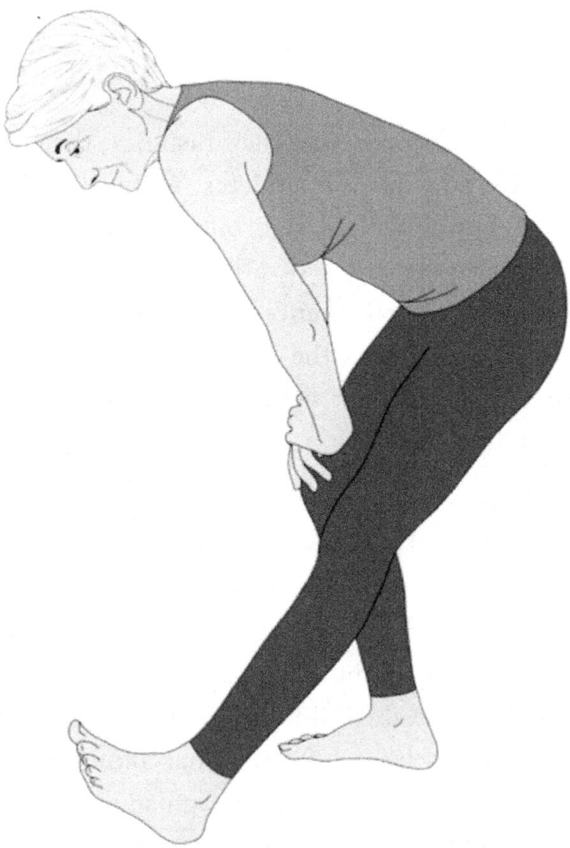

Fig 3.1 Standing Hamstring Stretch

Similarly, hip flexor strengthening exercises, such as lunges and leg raises, support the pelvis and lower back, crucial for maintaining proper form during athletic activities. A strong, flexible foundation helps prevent the overuse injuries that can sideline even the most dedicated athlete.

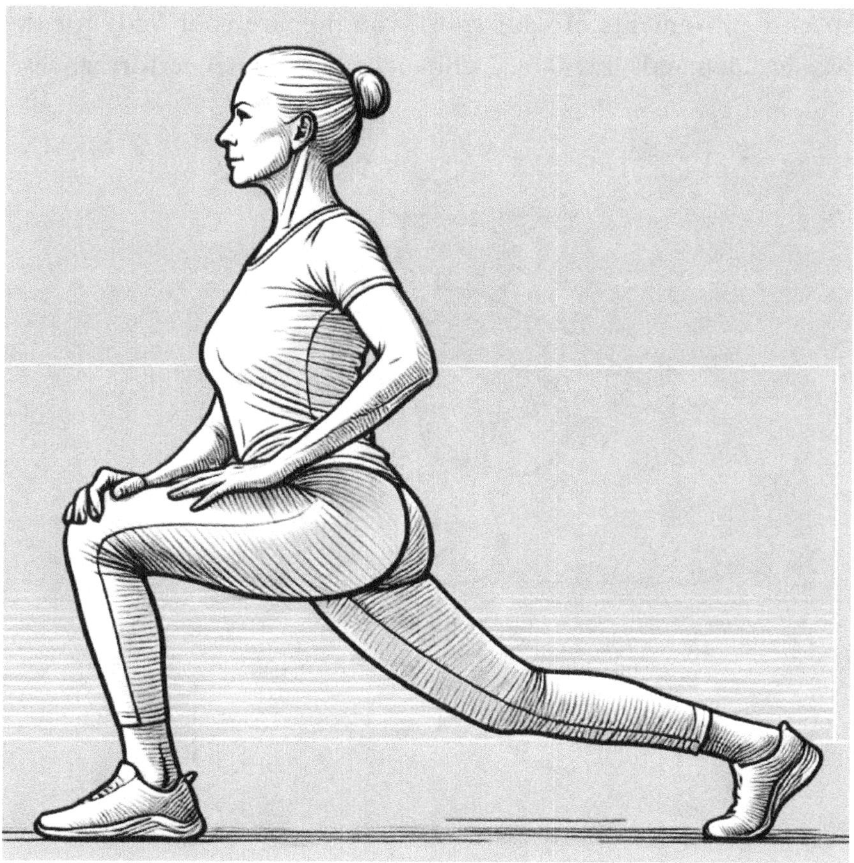

Fig 3.2 Lunge

Incorporating sport-specific movements into your training regimen tailors your preparation to the demands of your sport. Plyometric drills, for example, mimic the explosive movements used in sports like basketball and volleyball. These exercises, which include box jumps and burpees, condition the muscles for quick, powerful actions. They improve your ability to generate force rapidly, a key component in many athletic endeavors. Agility ladder exercises, on the other hand, enhance coordination and foot speed. These exercises are invaluable for sports requiring quick direction changes, such as football or tennis. By mimicking the specific movements of your sport, you prepare your body for the physical demands it will face, enhancing functional performance.

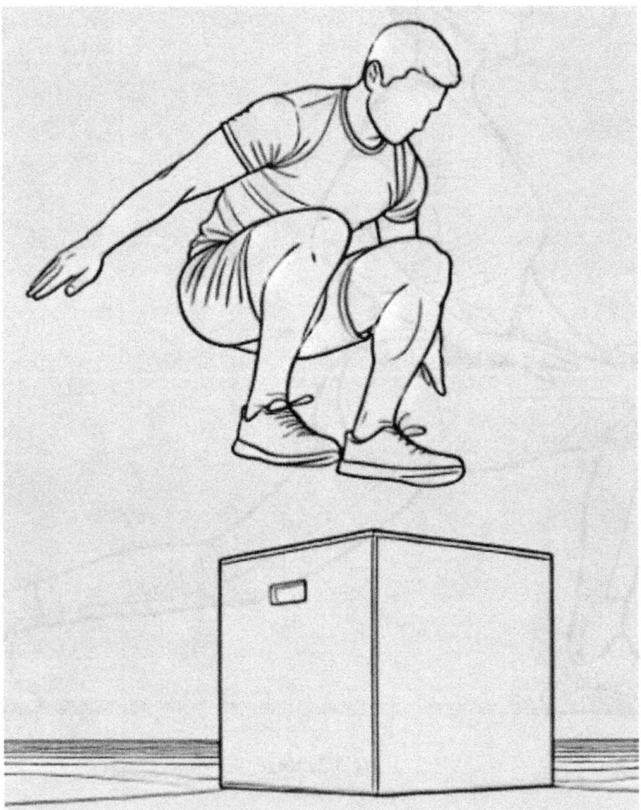

Fig 3.3 Box Jump

Recovery and cooldown routines are as vital as the workouts themselves. A well-structured cooldown helps transition your body from intense activity to rest, reducing the risk of muscle stiffness and soreness. Foam rolling is an effective technique to incorporate post-exercise. By applying pressure to specific areas of the body, foam rolling helps release muscle tightness, improving blood flow and aiding recovery. This self-myofascial release technique is a convenient way to enhance recovery at home or the gym. Complementing foam rolling with a yoga session provides a holistic approach to cooldown. Yoga stretches the muscles and calms the mind, offering a comprehensive recovery that addresses both physical and mental well-being.

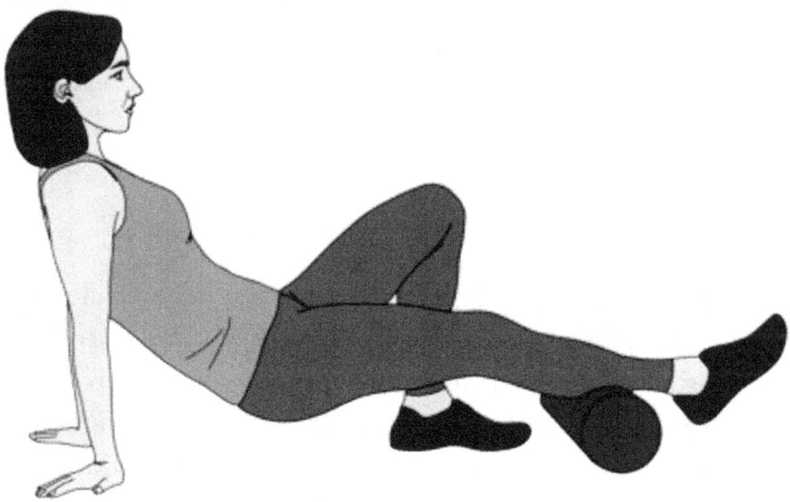

Fig 3.4 Foam Rolling Calf

Interactive Element: Create Your Recovery Routine

Developing a personalized recovery routine can optimize your athletic performance and prevent injury. Use this checklist to create a routine that fits your needs:

- **Daily Stretching**: Incorporate at least 10 minutes of stretching into your daily routine. Focus on key muscle groups like hamstrings and hip flexors.
- **Post-Workout Foam Rolling**: Spend 5-10 minutes foam rolling after workouts to relieve muscle tension.
- **Weekly Yoga Session**: Integrate a yoga session to enhance flexibility and promote mental relaxation.
- **Sport-Specific Drills**: Allocate time for plyometric drills and agility exercises tailored to your sport's demands.

These exercises form the backbone of a robust recovery strategy, ensuring athletes remain competitive while minimizing injury risk. Through deliberate practice and mindful recovery, athletes can sustain their performance, paving the way for success without compromising health.

3.1 YOUTH-FRIENDLY BACK CARE ROUTINES

Growing up in today's digital era presents unique challenges for youth, especially when it comes to back health. With screens becoming an integral part of daily life, many young individuals are developing poor posture from prolonged use of devices. Think about the hours spent hunched over tablets or phones, neck craned forward, shoulders slumped—a posture that, over time, can lead to discomfort and pain. The issue is compounded by growth-related pain, which is common during adolescence. As their bodies rapidly develop, young people may experience growing pains, particularly in the back, due to uneven growth spurts or increased physical activity. Early intervention is crucial in these formative years to prevent these habits from becoming lifelong issues.

To address these concerns, introducing fun and engaging exercises is key. Children and teenagers are more likely to stick with routines that feel less like exercise and more like play. Consider exercises such as animal walks, which mimic the movements of various animals. These not only engage the imagination but also encourage full-body coordination and strengthen muscles. Picture a group of kids moving like bears on all fours or hopping like frogs —each movement contributing to their back health in a playful manner.

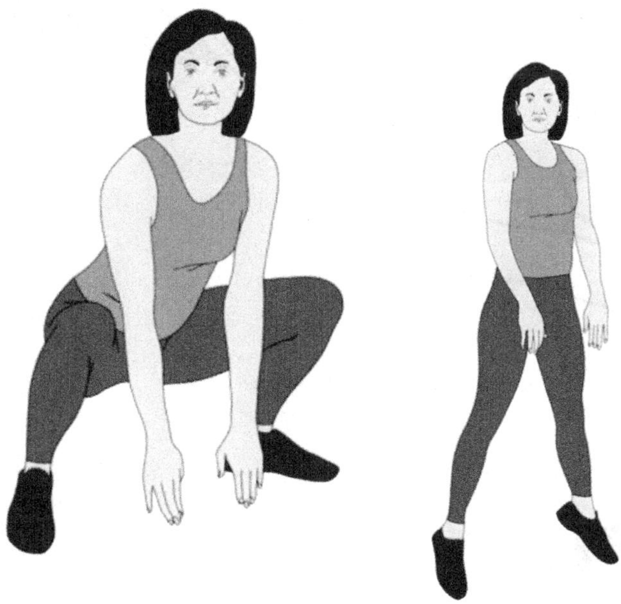

Fig 3.5 Frog Jumps

Dance-based workouts also offer a fantastic way to promote movement and flexibility. By combining rhythm and exercise, dance keeps young participants motivated and active. These activities can easily be adjusted to suit various skill levels, ensuring that all youth, regardless of their athleticism, can participate and benefit.

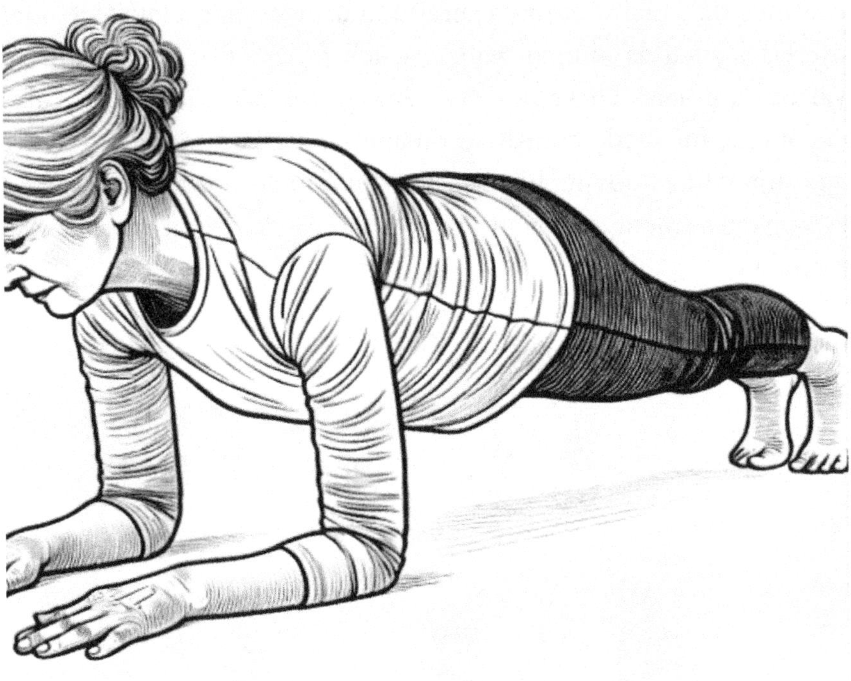

Fig 3.6 Plank

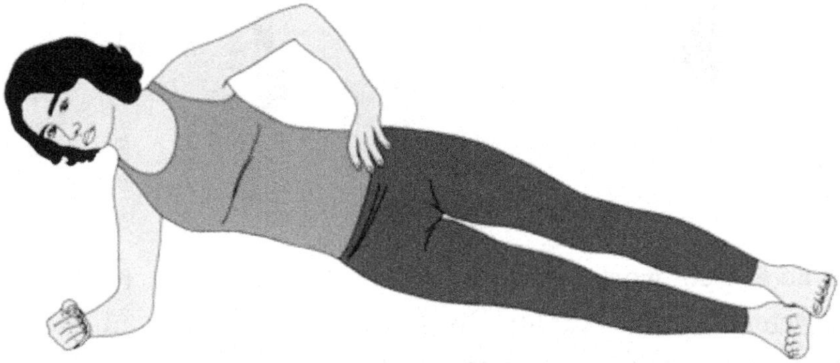

Fig 3.7 Plank Variation

Developing core strength early sets a strong foundation for preventing future back issues. The core, which includes the abdominal muscles, back muscles, and pelvis, acts as a stabilizing force for the spine. Exercises like plank variations are excellent for building this strength. By holding a plank position, youth engage multiple muscle groups, reinforcing the support structure for their spine.

Bicycle crunches, another effective exercise, target the abdominal muscles while promoting coordination. These exercises are straightforward yet effective, requiring no special equipment and can be done anywhere. Encouraging young individuals to incorporate these into their routines not only benefits their spine but also enhances their overall athletic ability.

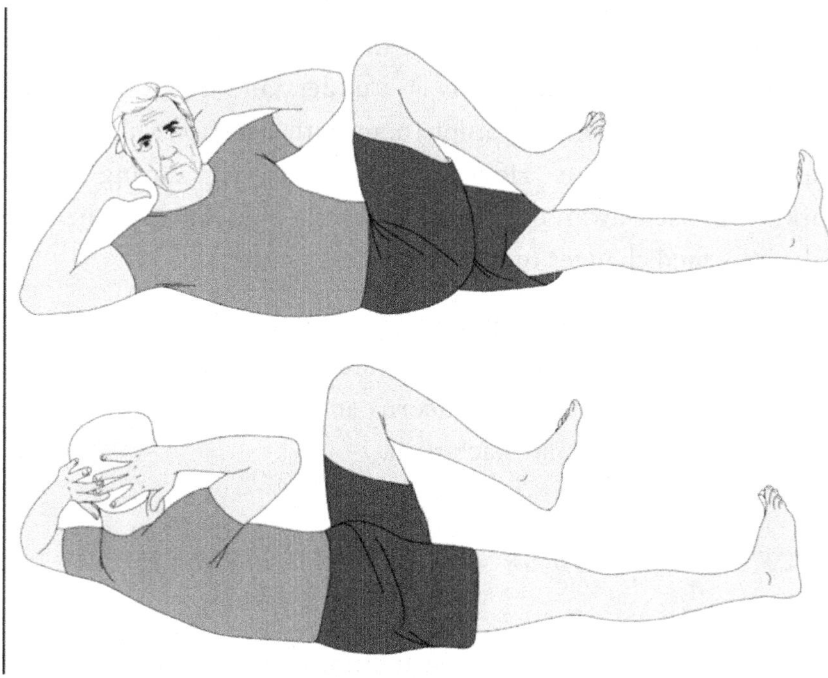

Fig 3.8 Bicycle Crunch

For parents and coaches, fostering an environment that supports healthy back practices is essential. Encouraging regular activity breaks, especially during long periods of study or screen time, can significantly reduce the risk of developing poor posture. Simple reminders to stand, stretch, or walk can refresh both body and mind. Monitoring posture during activities is another critical aspect. By teaching and reinforcing the importance of maintaining a neutral spine during various activities, adults can help youth develop lifelong habits that promote back health. This might involve gentle reminders to sit up straight, or demonstrating the correct way to carry a backpack to avoid unnecessary strain.

Reflection Section: Journaling for Youth

Encourage young people to keep a simple journal of their daily activities and any back discomfort they experience. This practice can help them identify patterns and understand how their habits affect their back health. Prompt them with questions like, "Did I take breaks today?" or "How did my posture feel during homework?" This self-awareness is a powerful tool, enabling them to make informed changes to their routines.

By addressing these issues with engaging and simple strategies, we can help guide today's youth towards healthier backs. These routines address immediate concerns and lay the groundwork for a future free from chronic back pain.

3.2 EXERCISES FOR SENIORS: LOW-IMPACT, HIGH-VALUE

In the later stages of life, maintaining mobility and strength becomes increasingly important, yet the approach must be gentle. High-intensity workouts are often unsuitable for seniors, as they can pose risks of injury and strain. Instead, focusing on low-impact exercises ensures that the body remains active without overexertion. Prioritizing safety and balance is essential, as these factors help prevent falls and maintain independence. Exercises that emphasize these elements allow seniors to build strength and confidence, enhancing their quality of life without unnecessary risk.

Balance and stability exercises are particularly crucial for seniors. These exercises not only improve physical stability, but also instill a sense of security when moving about. Standing leg lifts, for example, are simple yet effective. By standing tall and lifting one leg to the side, seniors engage muscles that support balance, reducing the likelihood of falls.

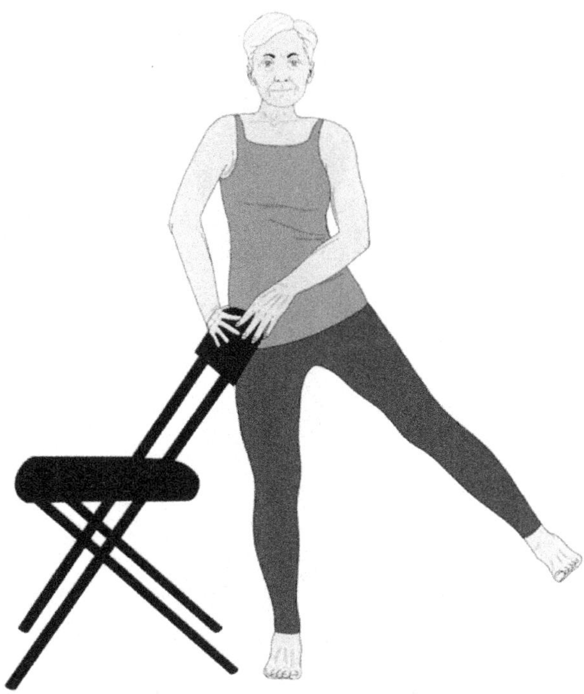

Fig 3.9 Standing Leg Lifts

Similarly, the heel-to-toe walk is another beneficial exercise. This involves walking in a straight line, placing the heel of one foot directly in front of the toes of the other. It's a small movement with significant benefits, as it hones coordination and balance, key components in preventing falls.

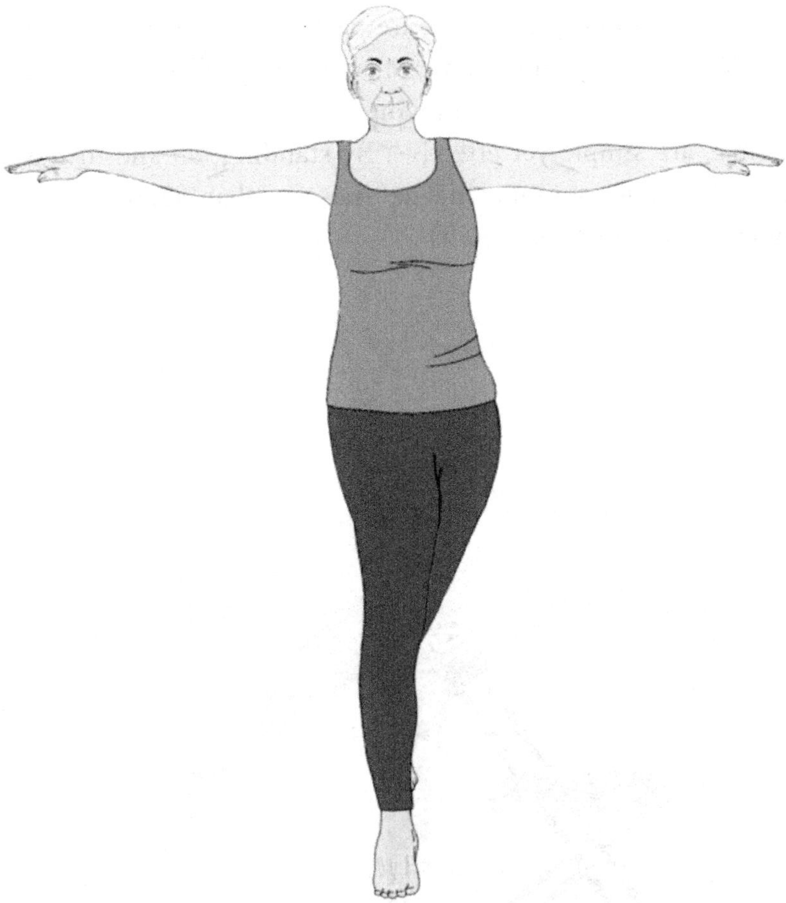

Fig 3.10 Heel to Toe Walk

Flexibility and joint mobility are vital for maintaining freedom of movement. Gentle stretches like Standing Hip Hinges offer a way to enhance flexibility without placing undue stress on the body. This exercise involves standing and pushing the hips backward helping to stretch the back and hamstrings. It's a soothing stretch that can be performed anywhere, providing relief and improved range of motion.

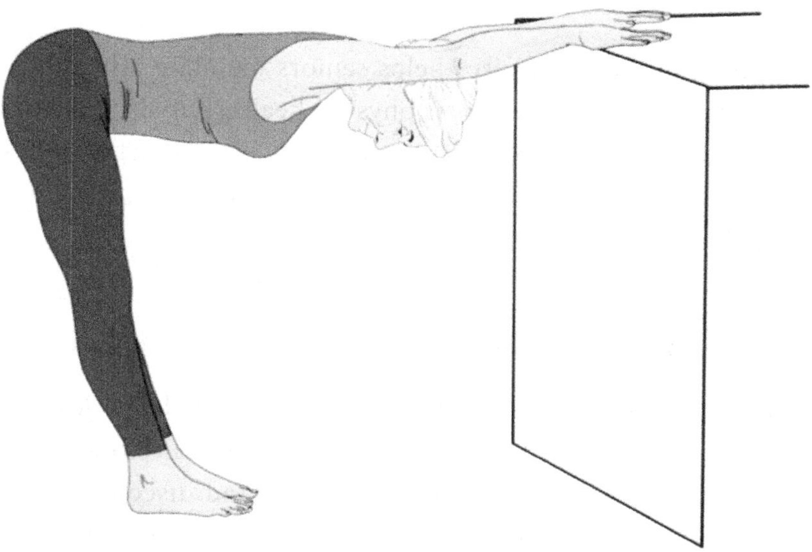

Fig 3.11 Standing Hip Hinge

Incorporating tai chi movements can further promote joint health. Tai chi, with its slow, deliberate actions, combines balance, flexibility, and strength training in a single practice. Its meditative nature also calms the mind, providing both physical and mental benefits, making it an excellent choice for seniors.

Group activities offer not only physical benefits but also social ones. Participating in group classes like chair yoga can provide seniors with motivation and camaraderie. Chair yoga adapts traditional yoga poses to a seated position, making it accessible to those with mobility limitations. The support of a chair allows seniors to safely explore movements that enhance flexibility and strength. Water aerobics sessions are another fantastic option. The buoyancy of water reduces impact on joints while providing resistance for muscle strengthening. These classes often foster a sense of community, encouraging regular participation and promoting social interaction.

Engaging in these exercises helps seniors maintain a healthy lifestyle, supporting not just their physical health, but also their social and emotional well-being. These activities are not just about exercise; they are about creating a life filled with vitality and connection.

3.3 TAILORING EXERCISES FOR DESK WORKERS

For many, the workday involves long hours seated at a desk, often without realizing the toll this takes on the back. Prolonged sitting compresses the spine, leading to stiffness and discomfort. It can also weaken the muscles meant to support your back, making you more susceptible to pain. The lack of movement reduces circulation, which is vital for maintaining muscle flexibility and joint lubrication. Over time, this sedentary lifestyle can contribute to conditions like chronic back pain or even more serious issues such as disc degeneration. To counteract these effects, regular movement breaks are crucial. Standing up and stretching every hour can do wonders for your back health, helping to reset posture and relieve pressure on the spine. Even brief walks to the water cooler or a quick jaunt around the office can break up the monotony of sitting, providing relief and promoting a healthier work environment.

Incorporating desk-friendly exercises into your routine can make a significant difference. These exercises are designed to be simple and convenient, allowing you to integrate them seamlessly into your workday. The seated spinal twist is a great example. While sitting, simply place your hand behind your hip, twisting your torso to look over your shoulder. Hold for a few breaths, feeling the stretch in your back and shoulders, then repeat on the other side.

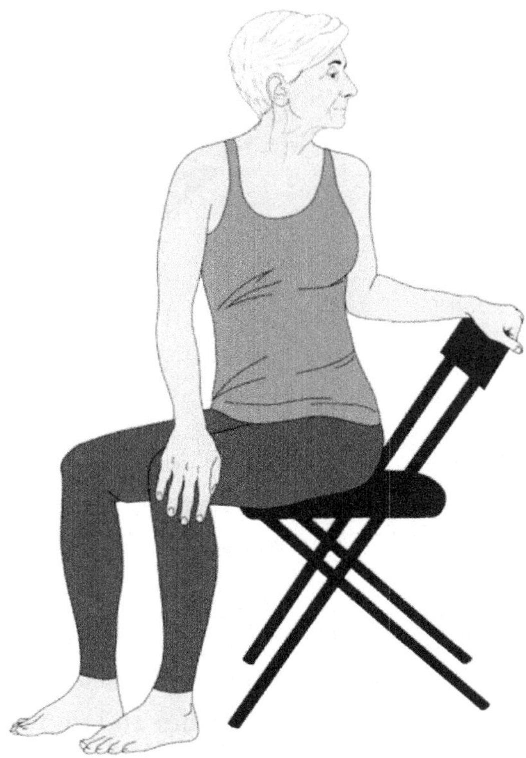

Fig 3.12 Sitting Spinal Twist

Another effective exercise is desk push-ups. Stand a few feet away from your desk, place your hands shoulder-width apart on its edge, and perform a push-up motion. This engages your chest and arms while giving your back a gentle stretch. Both exercises can be done in minutes and provide immediate benefits, enhancing flexibility and reducing tension.

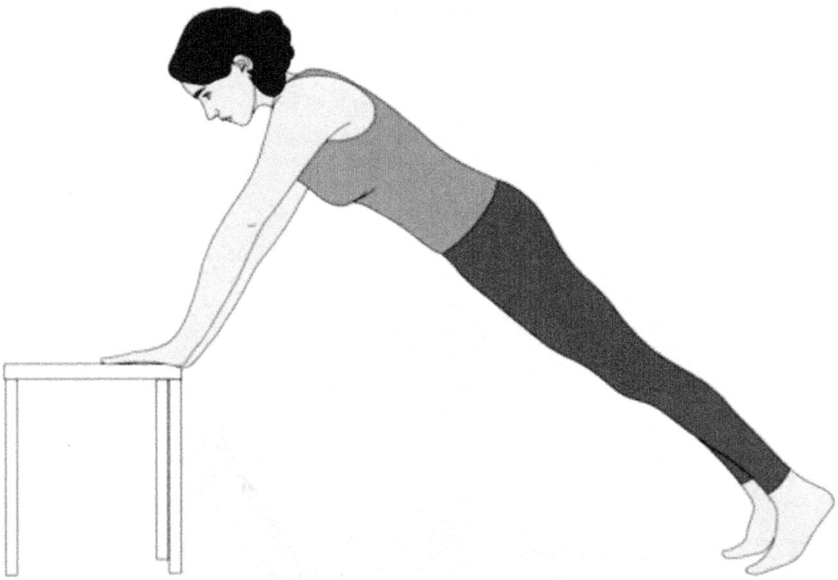

Fig 3.13 Desk Push-up

Posture correction is another key aspect of maintaining spine health at the desk. Over time, poor posture can lead to a host of issues, from muscle fatigue to headaches and, most notably, back pain. Exercises that target these problems can help mitigate them. Shoulder blade squeezes are a simple yet effective exercise. Sitting tall, draw your shoulder blades together and down, holding for a few seconds before releasing. This strengthens the muscles that support your upper back, promoting better posture.

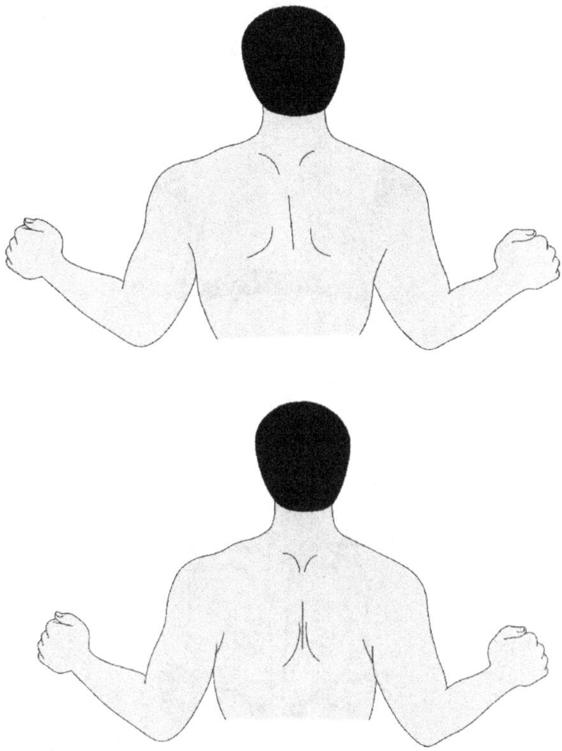

Fig 3.14 Sitting Shoulder Blade Squeeze

Chin tucks are equally important. While sitting or lying on your back, tuck your chin slightly and pull your head back over your shoulders. Hold this position briefly, then relax. These exercises, when practiced consistently, can significantly improve your posture, reducing the strain placed on your spine.

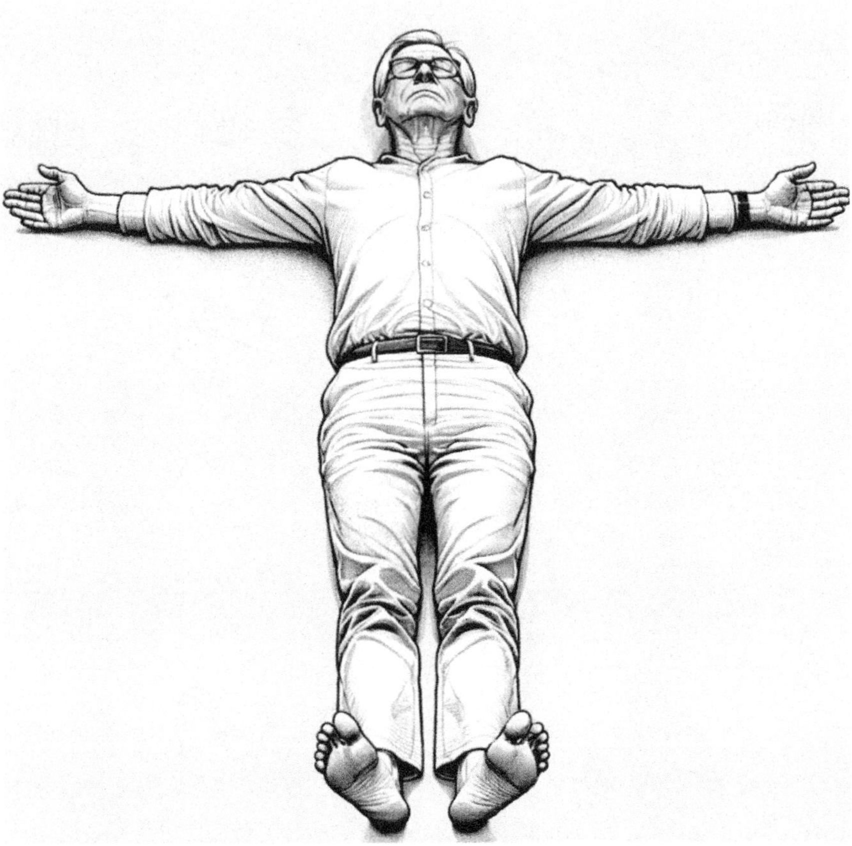

Fig 3.15 Lying Chin Tucks

A structured daily routine can help you maintain these practices throughout your workday. Start with a morning stretching session to prepare your body for the day ahead. Simple stretches like reaching for the sky or bending forward to touch your toes can invigorate your muscles and enhance your focus. Midday, take a mobility break. Stand up, move around, and perform a few desk-friendly exercises like the ones mentioned earlier. This benefits your back and refreshes your mind, making you more productive. By integrating these activities into your routine, you create a balanced approach to your workday, one that prioritizes your spine health alongside your professional responsibilities. These practices become a natural extension of your day, supporting a healthier, more comfortable you.

3.4 CORE STABILITY: STRENGTHENING THE SPINE'S SUPPORT SYSTEM

Consider your core as the foundation of your body's strength and stability. Comprised of muscles in the abdomen, lower back, and pelvis, these muscles act as a natural brace, stabilizing the spine and reducing the risk of injury. When your core is strong, it supports your spine, allowing you to maintain proper posture and balance. This stability is crucial, not just in sports or heavy lifting, but in everyday activities like walking, bending, or even sitting. A well-supported spine minimizes strain, preventing the back pain that so often results from poor posture or weak muscles. The benefits of a robust core extend beyond mere physical support; they enhance your ability to perform daily tasks with ease and comfort.

To achieve balanced core development, it's important to engage in exercises that target various core muscles. One effective exercise is the dead bug. Lying on your back, you lift your arms and legs towards the ceiling, then slowly lower one arm and the opposite leg towards the floor, keeping your back flat against the ground. This exercise engages multiple muscle groups, promoting coordination and stability.

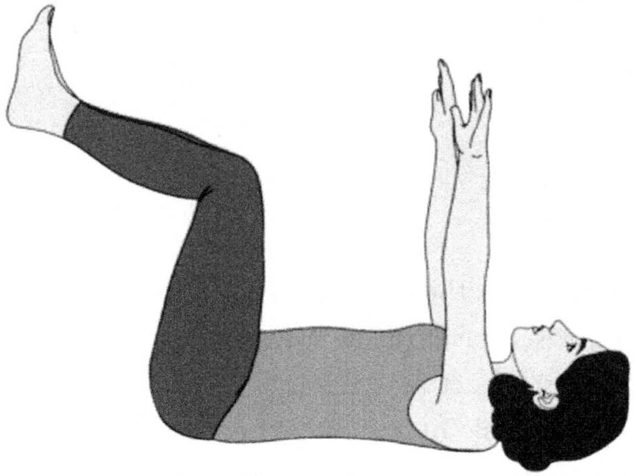

Fig 3.16 Dead Bug Start

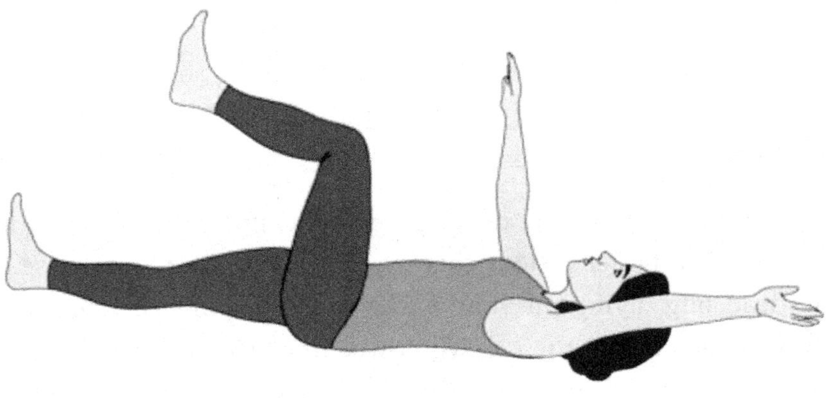

Fig 3.17 Dead Bug End

Another excellent core exercise is the Russian twist but should not be performed with active back pain. Seated with your feet elevated, you rotate your torso from side to side, touching the ground beside you. This movement strengthens the critical rotational oblique muscles. By incorporating these exercises into your routine, you ensure that all aspects of your core are addressed, fostering a well-rounded strength.

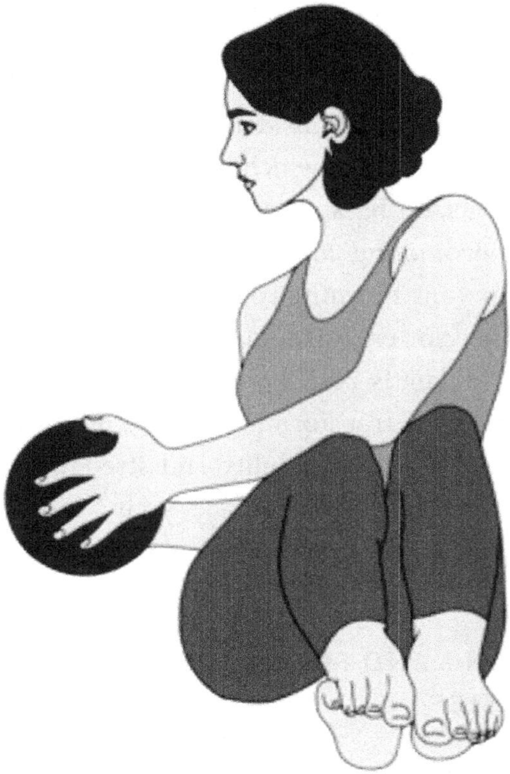

Fig 3.18 Sitting Russian Twist with Ball

Progression and safety are key when working on core stability. It's essential to start with exercises that match your current fitness level to prevent injury. Beginners might find it helpful to modify exercises to reduce intensity. For instance, if the dead bug is challenging, try performing it without lowering your limbs as far, or keep your knees bent. As your strength improves, gradually increase the difficulty by extending your limbs further or adding resistance, such as holding a small weight during Russian twists. Maintaining proper form is crucial for effectiveness and safety. Focus on controlled movements, ensuring your back remains flat and your core engaged. This focus on form prevents strain and maximizes the benefits of your efforts.

Incorporating core exercises into your daily routine helps ensure continuous improvement. Consider adding core circuits to your gym sessions. These circuits, which involve performing a series of core exercises back-to-back, keep your workouts dynamic and engaging while promoting core endurance. Alternatively, include core exercises in your morning routine. A few minutes of planks or Russian twists can energize you for the day ahead, setting a positive tone. The key is consistency; regular practice reinforces strength and stability, transforming these exercises from a task into a habit. Over time, the stability and strength gained from a dedicated core routine will enhance your overall well-being, providing the support your spine needs to thrive.

3.5 STRETCHING AND FLEXIBILITY: KEY MOVEMENTS FOR PAIN RELIEF

Flexibility plays a crucial role in managing back pain, offering a path towards enhanced mobility and reduced discomfort. When your muscles are flexible, they can move more freely, which significantly diminishes tension. This reduced tension lessens the strain on your spine, allowing you to move with greater ease. Imagine the freedom of being able to bend, stretch, and twist without that familiar twinge of pain. Regular stretching not only alleviates current discomfort but also fortifies your body against future episodes of pain. Over time, maintaining a routine of flexibility exercises can lead to improved posture, better balance, and a more resilient musculoskeletal system. The long-term benefits of regular stretching are profound, contributing to overall well-being and a more active lifestyle.

Incorporating various stretching techniques into your daily regimen can provide targeted relief and promote relaxation. Understanding the differences between dynamic and static stretching is key. Dynamic stretching involves controlled, gentle movements that prepare your muscles for activity. These stretches are particularly useful as a warm-up, gradually increasing your range of motion and circulation. Consider leg swings or arm circles before embarking on a workout, gently coaxing your muscles into readiness.

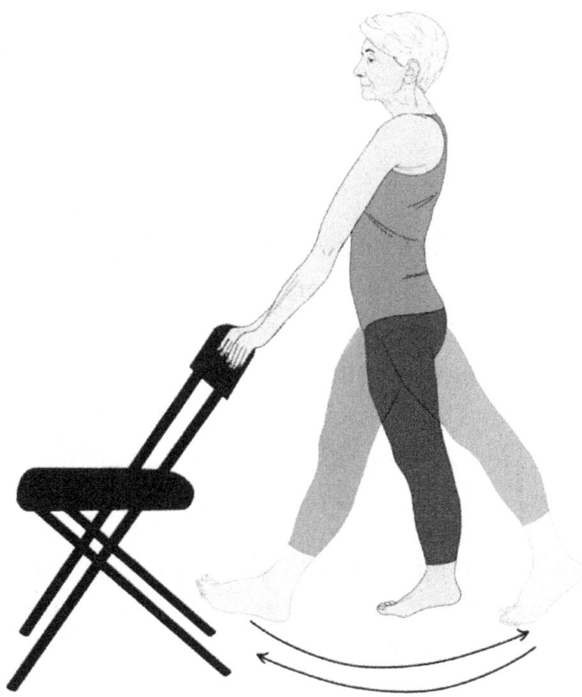

Fig 3.19 Leg Swings

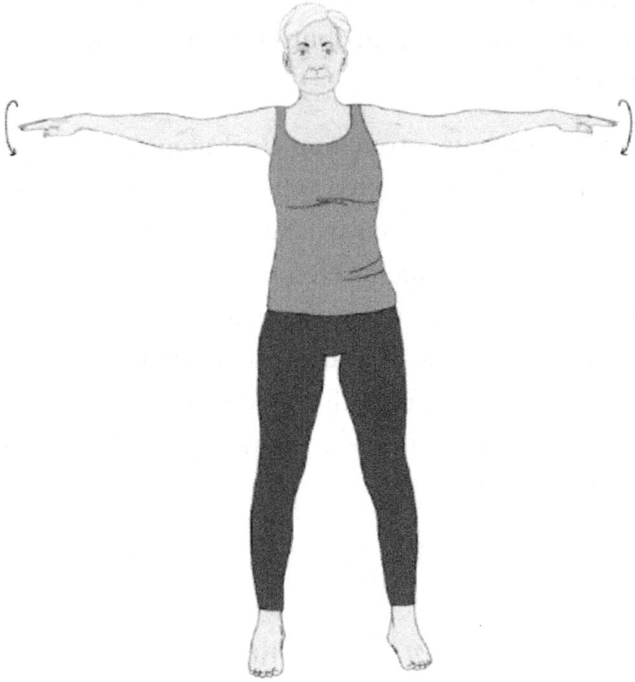

Fig 3.20 Arm Circles

In contrast, static stretching involves holding a position for a prolonged period, typically after physical activity. This technique helps elongate muscles and alleviate tension. Imagine reaching for your toes and holding the position, feeling the gradual release of tightness in your legs and lower back. Passive stretching, another effective method, uses external forces like gravity or a partner to deepen the stretch, offering a more intense release without active effort.

Establishing stretching routines tailored to different times of the day can enhance their effectiveness. Morning routines should focus on energizing stretches that awaken your body and prepare you for the day ahead. Simple movements, such as reaching for the sky can invigorate your muscles and clear the mental fog. These exercises increase blood flow and stimulate your nervous system, setting a positive tone for the hours to come.

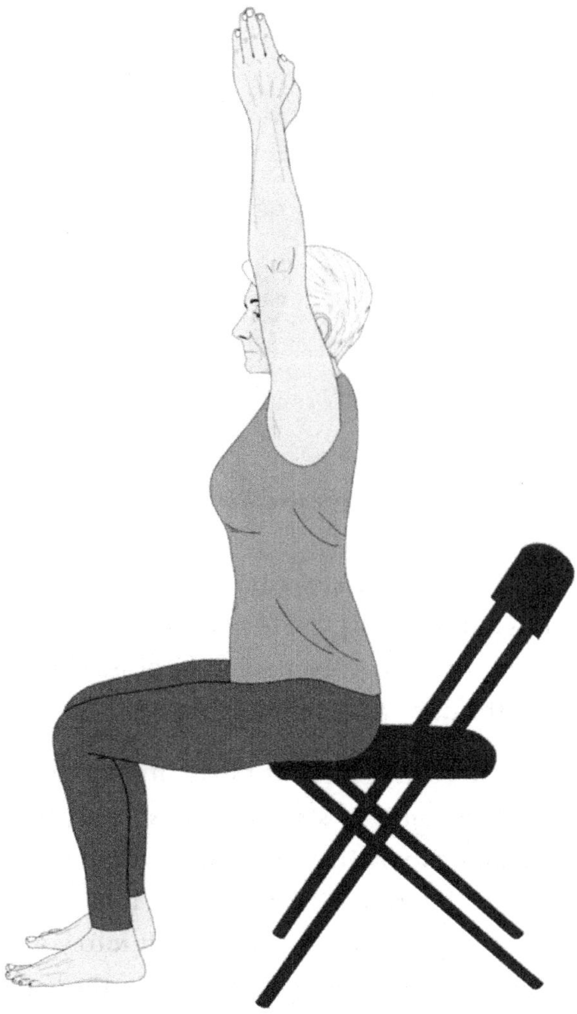

Fig 3.21 Reaching for the Sky

Throughout the day, incorporating brief stretching sessions can relieve stress and prevent stiffness. Consider taking a few moments to perform shoulder rolls or standing neck stretches during work breaks, counteracting the effects of prolonged sitting.

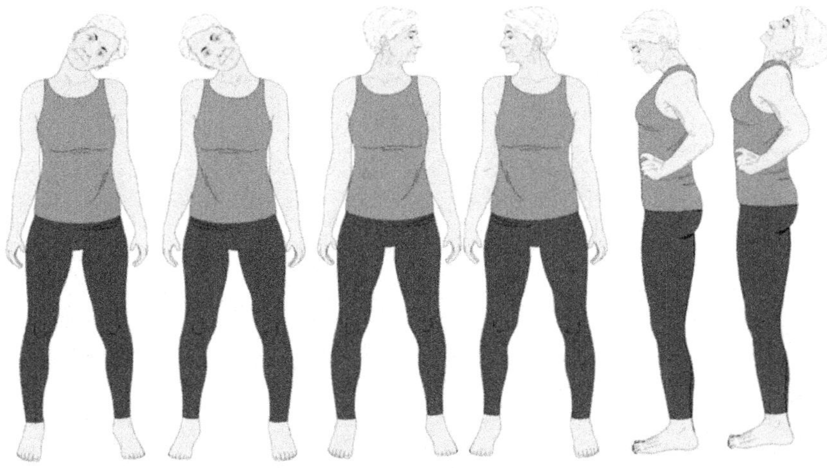

Fig 3.22 Standing Neck Stretches

As evening approaches, relaxation stretches become valuable, helping to unwind and prepare for restful sleep. Gentle forward bends or seated stretches promote calmness, encouraging your body to release the day's accumulated tension.

Consistency is the cornerstone of flexibility and pain prevention. Establishing a daily habit of stretching ensures that your muscles remain supple and supportive. It's about weaving stretching into the fabric of your life, rather than viewing it as a chore. Whether you set aside time each morning, integrate it into your workout, or use it as a transitional moment between tasks, the key is regularity. Over time, these small, consistent efforts yield significant results, fostering a more flexible and resilient body. This commitment to consistency strengthens the mind-body connection, empowering you to take control of your physical well-being.

As we wrap up this chapter on exercise programs, remember that each movement you make contributes to your overall health. Stretching is not just about easing back pain; it's about enhancing your quality of life. By embracing these practices, you create a foundation of strength and flexibility that supports all your activities. Next, we will explore more about how lifestyle choices intertwine with physical health, revealing opportunities for lasting improvement.

4

EMBRACING TECHNOLOGY AND MODERN SOLUTIONS

In the fast-paced world we live in today, technology has become an integral part of our daily lives, permeating every aspect, from how we communicate to how we manage our health. It's fascinating to observe how these advancements have revolutionized the way we approach well-being, particularly in the realm of back health. For many, the journey toward a healthier spine often begins with the simple tap of a button on a smartphone. Fitness apps, once a novelty, now stand as powerful tools in the fight against back pain, offering structure and accountability that were once only achievable through in-person consultations. They transform the often daunting process of recovery into a manageable, even engaging, experience where progress is not just hoped for but meticulously tracked and celebrated.

Fitness apps provide a structured approach to recovery by offering goal-setting and progress-tracking features that keep you motivated and on course. These digital platforms allow you to set specific, measurable objectives, whether it's improving flexibility, increasing core strength, or simply committing to regular exercise.

As you log each workout and tick off milestones, the sense of accomplishment fuels further dedication. The customizable workout plans cater to your individual needs, accommodating your current fitness level and gradually increasing in intensity as you progress. This adaptability ensures that you remain challenged without feeling overwhelmed, making the path to recovery both achievable and sustainable.

Among the myriad of fitness apps available, a few stand out for their user-friendliness and effectiveness in promoting back health. MyFitnessPal, renowned for its comprehensive nutrition tracking, helps you make informed dietary choices that support overall health and spine wellness. By logging your meals, you gain insights into your nutritional intake, identifying areas for improvement and ensuring you fuel your body with the right nutrients. Strava, on the other hand, is a favorite among athletes for its robust activity logging features. It tracks your workouts, providing detailed analytics on performance and encouraging friendly competition with its social features. For those seeking personalized workout routines, Fitbod offers tailored plans that adapt as you log your progress, ensuring each session aligns with your goals and current capabilities.

The integration of fitness apps with other technologies amplifies their benefits, creating a seamless health monitoring experience. Many apps sync effortlessly with smartwatches, transferring data like steps taken, calories burned, and even sleep patterns. This integration allows for a comprehensive overview of your activity levels, providing insights that inform your recovery approach. By connecting with heart rate monitors, these apps deliver real-time feedback on your exertion levels, ensuring you exercise within safe and effective parameters. This interconnectedness enhances the functionality of each device and empowers you with a holistic view of your health metrics, making adjustments as necessary to optimize your progress.

Choosing the right app requires careful consideration of your individual goals and preferences. Start by researching user reviews and ratings to gauge the app's reliability and effectiveness. Look for apps that offer features specific to back health, such as exercises designed to strengthen the core and improve posture. The availability of instructional videos or guided sessions can also be a valuable resource, providing visual cues and techniques to ensure proper form and prevent injury. Additionally, consider whether the app's interface is intuitive and easy to navigate, as a user-friendly design encourages regular use and enhances your overall experience.

Interactive Element: App Selection Checklist

- **Define Your Goals**: Clarify what you hope to achieve with the app—be it flexibility, strength, or pain management.
- **Check Reviews and Ratings**: Look for user feedback on app performance and effectiveness.
- **Assess Features**: Ensure the app includes specific exercises and tracking tools relevant to back health.
- **Ease of Use**: Evaluate the app's interface for simplicity and accessibility.
- **Integration Options**: Consider if the app syncs with other devices you use for a comprehensive health approach.

Engaging with fitness apps is more than a modern convenience; it's a strategic step in managing and preventing back pain. By leveraging the capabilities of these digital tools, you take an active role in your health journey, transforming your smartphone into a personal trainer, nutritionist, and motivator, all in one. Through careful selection and consistent use, these apps can be a cornerstone in your strategy for achieving and maintaining a healthy, pain-free back.

4.1 ONLINE RESOURCES: FINDING RELIABLE INFORMATION

In today's digital age, the internet is a vast ocean of information, some of it credible, some not. Navigating this space, especially when it comes to health, requires a discerning eye. The importance of accessing accurate, evidence-based information for managing back health cannot be overstated. Imagine setting out on a road trip without a reliable map—you're bound to get lost. The same applies to your health journey; you need a trusted guide. Checking the credibility of your sources is paramount. Look for websites that are backed by reputable health organizations or peer-reviewed studies. These sites often provide the most reliable information, vetted by experts who know their field inside and out. Credibility ensures that the advice you follow is not just anecdotal but grounded in science.

Identifying reputable health websites is your first line of defense against misinformation. The Mayo Clinic's website is a goldmine for reliable medical information, known for its comprehensive articles that cover a range of health topics, including back pain. Similarly, WebMD's back pain section offers valuable insights into symptoms, treatments, and preventive measures, often reviewed by medical professionals. Another excellent resource is Healthline, where expert-reviewed articles provide clarity and depth on various health issues. These platforms are not only trustworthy but also user-friendly, enabling anyone to understand complex medical concepts without feeling overwhelmed. They serve as a guide, offering well-researched information that can help inform your decisions about back health.

The internet is rife with misinformation, a potential minefield for those seeking health advice. Sensationalized content, often designed to attract clicks rather than inform, can lead you astray. Recognizing these pitfalls is crucial. Be wary of articles that make grandiose claims without supporting evidence, or those that promote miracle cures. Such content often lacks the scrutiny of qualified experts. Unverified health claims can be dangerous, leading to practices that might worsen your condition or delay appropriate treatment. To protect yourself, cross-reference information with multiple sources, and always err on the side of caution when encountering dubious advice.

For those eager to deepen their understanding of back health, online courses offer structured learning experiences that go beyond what typical websites provide. Platforms like Coursera offer courses in anatomy and physiology, providing foundational knowledge that can enhance your understanding of how the body works. These courses, often led by university professors, offer a chance to learn from experts in the field. Similarly, Udemy provides classes on exercise science, where you can explore the mechanics of movement and how to optimize it for your spine's benefit. Enrolling in these courses empowers you to take control of your learning, equipping you with the knowledge to make informed decisions about your health.

Resource List: Trusted Online Platforms for Back Health Information

- **Mayo Clinic**: Comprehensive medical information and back pain insights.

- **WebMD**: Detailed health guides and expert-reviewed content.
- **Healthline**: In-depth articles on symptoms, treatments, and prevention.

In the vast expanse of online information, these resources stand out as beacons of reliability. By focusing on credible sources and engaging in structured learning, you can navigate the digital landscape with confidence, making informed choices that support your journey to better back health.

4.2 POSTURE CHECK 3D™ FROM FOOT LEVELERS

In our modern lives, where we are often glued to screens and seated for long stretches, maintaining proper posture has become a significant challenge. It's not just about aesthetics; poor posture can lead to a cascade of health issues, including persistent back pain, neck strain, and even headaches. The Posture Check 3D™ from Foot Levelers offers a cutting-edge solution to this pervasive problem, providing a detailed analysis that goes far beyond the superficial. Imagine being able to measure and understand the intricacies of your posture with precision. This innovative tool utilizes advanced technology to deliver insights that can transform how you approach your spine health.

The 3D Posture Scanner is an integral part of this system. It provides analytical measurements of forward head posture, known as the Tech Neck Index™, a condition exacerbated by prolonged device use. This measurement is crucial because even a slight forward tilt of the head can significantly increase the strain on the neck and upper back muscles. By understanding the degree of this posture deviation, you can take targeted steps to correct it, such as adjusting your workspace or incorporating specific exercises to strengthen the neck and shoulder muscles. The scanner's precision offers a clear picture of how your posture might be contributing to back pain and other discomforts, empowering you to make changes that have a real impact.

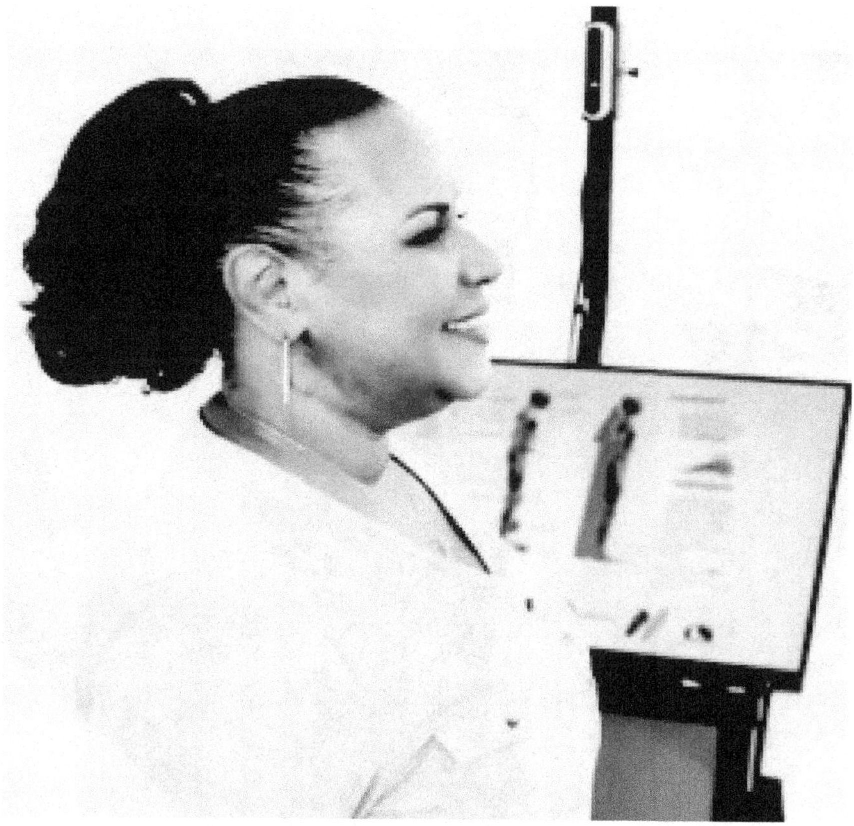

Fig 4.1 3D Posture Scanner

Complementing this is the 3D Foot Scanner, which highlights imbalances and asymmetries between the feet using the Pronation Stability Index™. The feet are the foundation of our body, and any imbalance in this area can ripple upwards, affecting posture and contributing to back pain. This scanner assesses the status of all three arches of the foot, providing a comprehensive view of how these structures support your body. If your feet are not properly aligned, it can lead to compensatory adjustments in your posture, increasing the risk of pain and injury. By identifying these imbalances, the 3D Foot Scanner enables you to address them, whether through custom orthotics or exercises designed to enhance foot stability.

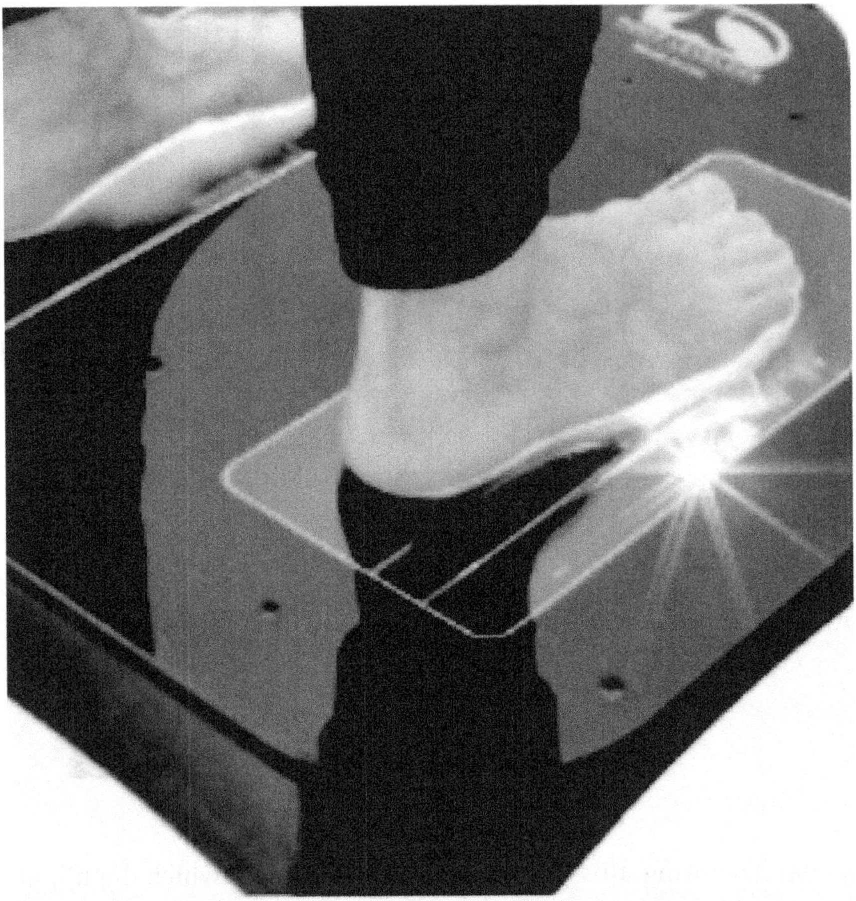

Fig 4.2 3D Foot Scanner

An added feature is the Stability Assessment Recommendation Assistant, or SARA, which offers personalized product recommendations based on a simple survey. This assistant analyzes your posture data and suggests interventions tailored to your specific needs. SARA provides guidance that is directly relevant to your posture and lifestyle. These recommendations make it easier to implement changes that will have the most significant impact on your spinal health, ensuring that you are not just treating symptoms but addressing the root causes of your discomfort.

The Posture Check 3D™ system culminates in a Report of Findings, offering a full-body analysis from head to toe. This comprehensive report is not merely a collection of data points; it is a roadmap for improving your posture and, by extension, your overall health. By detailing where specific issues lie, the report helps you understand the interconnectedness of your body's alignment. With this knowledge, you can make informed decisions about your health, whether it's choosing to consult a specialist, adjusting your daily habits, or investing in supportive products.

For athletes, adults, and youth alike, the Posture Check 3D™ is a valuable tool in the quest for optimal health. It provides the insights needed to understand how posture affects your body, offering actionable data that can guide your efforts to improve alignment and reduce pain. Whether you're looking to enhance athletic performance, prevent future injuries, or simply live without the nagging discomfort of poor posture, this technology offers a clear path forward. It bridges the gap between awareness and action, transforming how you approach your spine health with precision and confidence. To get a complimentary Posture Check 3D™ and 3D Foot Scan, simply find a location near you here:

https://www.footlevelers.com/about/find-a-healthcare-provider-near-you?utm_source=PC3D

4.3 WEARABLE TECH: MONITORING YOUR HEALTH IN REAL-TIME

In an age where information is at our fingertips, wearable technology has emerged as a trusted companion in navigating the nuances of personal health. Devices like smartwatches and fitness trackers have transcended their status as mere gadgets, evolving into essential tools for monitoring various health metrics. At the core of these wearables is the ability to track steps and activity levels, providing a clear picture of your daily movement. But they do more than count steps. They measure heart rate, offering insights into cardiovascular health, and monitor sleep patterns to help you understand how well you rest. This data is invaluable, shedding light on areas that might need attention and providing a roadmap for improvement.

For individuals focusing on back health, wearables offer specific benefits that align with the goals of recovery and prevention. Real-time data from these devices empowers you to make informed decisions about your physical activity and recovery progress. Alerts for prolonged inactivity serve as gentle reminders to move, breaking up long periods of sitting that can exacerbate back pain. The feedback on sleep quality is crucial, especially since poor sleep can affect pain perception and recovery. By identifying patterns in your sleep and activity, wearables enable you to adjust your lifestyle in ways that promote spine health, ensuring you are moving enough and resting well.

Several wearable devices have become popular for their effectiveness in tracking health metrics related to back health. The Fitbit, renowned for its comprehensive activity tracking, provides detailed insights into your daily movements and sleep patterns. It acts as a constant companion, encouraging you to stay active and maintain a healthy routine. On the other hand, the Apple Watch integrates health features seamlessly, offering not just fitness tracking, but also heart rate monitoring and even ECG capabilities. It provides reminders to stand, breathe, and move throughout the day, all of which contribute to maintaining a healthy back. These devices are more than just accessories; they are integrated health tools that support your journey towards a pain-free life.

Integrating wearables into your daily life can maximize their potential and enhance your health monitoring efforts. Setting daily movement goals is a practical way to ensure you remain active, even on busy days. Whether it's reaching a certain step count or achieving a specific activity level, these goals keep you motivated and focused. Utilizing health apps linked to wearables can further enrich your experience. Many apps offer personalized insights, suggesting adjustments based on your data and helping you track progress over time. They provide a platform for setting goals, viewing trends, and even connecting with friends for added motivation. By embracing these technologies, you transform your approach to health, taking proactive steps to maintain and improve your back health.

4.4 VIRTUAL COACHING: ACCESSING EXPERTISE FROM ANYWHERE

In today's interconnected world, the barriers of geography have all but vanished, opening up a realm of possibilities for accessing professional expertise right from the comfort of your home. Virtual coaching has emerged as a game-changer in the fitness and rehabilitation sectors, offering personalized guidance that was once confined to in-person sessions. Through online platforms, you can now connect with expert coaches who provide tailored workout plans and real-time feedback, ensuring your exercises are effective and safe. This level of personalization was difficult to come by in traditional settings, where time and location constraints often limited access to specialized care. Now, whether you're in a bustling city or a remote village, the world's best coaches are just a click away, ready to help you achieve your health goals.

One of the standout benefits of virtual coaching is the flexibility it offers. Unlike traditional coaching, where schedules must align perfectly, virtual sessions allow you to choose times that fit your lifestyle. This adaptability means you can incorporate your fitness routine into your day without the hassle of commuting or rearranging other commitments. With regular check-ins and progress reviews, virtual coaches ensure that you stay on track, holding you accountable while providing the motivation needed to push through challenging phases. The digital format also allows for frequent communication, whether through video calls, emails, or messaging, creating a support system that adapts to your needs and preferences. This constant interaction fosters a sense of trust and collaboration between you and your coach, crucial for sustained motivation.

Selecting the right virtual coach involves more than just a quick internet search. It's important to consider several factors to ensure the coach aligns with your personal recovery goals and needs. Start by evaluating their credentials and experience, particularly in back health, to verify their expertise. A coach with a solid background in rehabilitation or sports science is more likely to understand the complexities of your condition and provide effective solutions. Compatibility is another key aspect. Consider how you prefer to communicate—whether through detailed emails, quick text messages, or video calls—and ensure your coach is comfortable with these methods. The right coach will not only have the credentials but will also communicate in a way that resonates with you, making the process smoother and more enjoyable.

Several platforms have made it easier than ever to connect with qualified coaches and trainers. Trainerize, for instance, offers custom fitness programs that can be tailored to your specific needs and goals. This platform allows coaches to track your progress and make adjustments to your plan as needed, ensuring you get the most out of each session. Another popular platform, Noom, takes a holistic approach to health coaching, focusing not just on physical activity but also on nutrition and behavioral changes. With Noom, you gain access to a comprehensive support system that helps you develop healthier habits, providing a well-rounded approach to your health journey. These platforms are designed to be user-friendly, making it easy for you to navigate your fitness journey with confidence and clarity.

The rise of virtual coaching represents a significant shift in how we approach fitness and rehabilitation, making expert guidance accessible to a wider audience. Whether you're an athlete looking to optimize performance, an adult seeking to alleviate chronic pain, or a youth aiming to develop healthy habits, virtual coaching offers the tools and support you need to succeed. By harnessing the power of technology, you can engage with top-tier coaches who bring a wealth of knowledge and experience to your screen, guiding you toward a healthier, more active lifestyle.

4.5 SOCIAL MEDIA COMMUNITIES: SUPPORT AND SHARED EXPERIENCES

In a world where technology bridges the gap between individuals across continents, social media communities have emerged as vital support systems for those grappling with back pain. These online groups offer more than just a platform to share stories; they create a sense of belonging among individuals who might otherwise feel isolated in their struggles. When you join these communities, you tap into a wellspring of emotional encouragement from peers who truly understand your experiences. It's a place where sharing a small victory, like completing a pain-free day or discovering a new exercise, is met with genuine celebration. Such interactions foster a positive environment, making the path to recovery feel less daunting and more achievable.

The benefits of participating in these communities extend beyond emotional support. They serve as a hub for exchanging tips and success stories, offering practical advice that you can incorporate into your daily life. By engaging with others, you gain access to a diverse array of perspectives and solutions that might not have crossed your mind. This collective wisdom is invaluable, providing fresh insights and alternative approaches to managing back pain. Whether it's a new stretching technique, advice on ergonomic adjustments, or recommendations for local healthcare professionals, the shared knowledge within these communities can be transformative. The sense of camaraderie and motivation found in these groups can reignite your determination to pursue a healthier lifestyle.

Engaging in social media groups requires a mindful approach to ensure interactions remain positive and beneficial for all members. Respectful and supportive communication forms the backbone of these communities, encouraging open dialogue and fostering a safe space for everyone to share their experiences. It's crucial to avoid spreading misinformation or unverified advice, as these can lead to confusion or harm. Instead, focus on sharing personal experiences and verified information, always mindful of the impact your words might have on others. By maintaining a respectful tone and supporting fellow members, you contribute to a constructive environment that uplifts rather than undermines.

Several social media platforms host active and supportive back pain communities. Facebook, with its vast user base, offers numerous support groups dedicated to chronic pain management. These groups often have moderators who ensure discussions remain on track and that the information shared is reliable. Similarly, Reddit hosts forums where users can engage in candid discussions about their struggles and triumphs. These forums, known for their diverse user base, provide a wealth of firsthand experiences and advice. By exploring these platforms, you can find a community that resonates with your needs and preferences, offering both support and practical solutions.

As you immerse yourself in these online communities, you'll discover a network of individuals who share your challenges and victories. Together, you can navigate the complexities of back pain, drawing strength and inspiration from shared experiences. This chapter has highlighted how technology can enhance your journey to better back health, providing tools and communities that support your efforts. Embrace these resources as you continue to explore ways to improve your well-being, knowing that you're not alone on this path.

REDUCING BACK PAIN ON A LARGER SCALE

"The end of all knowledge should be service to others."

— CESAR CHAVEZ

Experts estimate that the number of people suffering from lower back pain will increase steadily over the coming years, reaching 843 million people by 2050 (World Health Organization 2023). The reason for the increase is population growth and aging, and although this makes sense, it means that it's more important than ever to equip people with the tools and information they need to relieve their pain.

While an aging population may be part of the reason that we're seeing an increase in the number of cases of lower back pain, it affects a great many younger people, too, and when we can take steps to address it early on, it's less likely to be a problem later in life. In my work as a sports chiropractor, I saw many cases that could have seriously hampered someone's athletic career had they not been dealt with, and when I retired, I knew that my work wasn't done. There's so much people can do to take control of their own back health when they have the right tools, and I'm honored to be in a position to share my expertise through writing.

My mission is to help as many people as I can manage their own back pain and make the lifestyle changes necessary to achieve long-term back health. And maybe, just maybe, if enough people acquire that knowledge, we might be able to stop the number of cases from reaching 843 million by 2050. As you might have guessed, this is where I'd like to ask for your help. I can reach more people with this information if you'd be willing to spread the word, and the good news is, you can do that simply by leaving a short review.

By leaving a review of this book on Amazon, you'll make it easier for other people to find it, and as a result, more people will have the tools they need to take charge of their back health.

Reviews help people find the information they're looking for and tell them about other people's experiences with the books that have helped them. Your review could be a huge help to other people currently suffering from lower back pain.

Thank you so much for your support. Together, I know we can make a real difference.

Scan the QR code below.

5

RECOVERY PROTOCOLS AND PROGRESS TRACKING

Imagine standing at the base of a mountain, gazing at the peak, knowing the journey ahead is both daunting and exhilarating. Recovery from lower back pain can feel much the same. It requires determination, a clear plan, and the right tools to navigate each step of the way. The path to healing is not a one-size-fits-all endeavor; it demands a customized approach that considers your unique needs and circumstances. This chapter serves as your map, guiding you through the phases of recovery with clarity and purpose.

At the heart of any successful recovery plan is an initial assessment and baseline setting. This crucial first step involves evaluating your current condition, identifying pain triggers, and understanding your physical limitations. It's akin to charting the starting point on your mountain climb, giving you a clear picture of where you stand before embarking on the ascent. This assessment provides the foundation on which your entire recovery plan is built, ensuring that each subsequent step is tailored to your individual needs. Whether you're an athlete pushing for peak performance or an office worker seeking relief from chronic discomfort, understanding your baseline is essential for progress.

With your baseline established, the next phase is the introduction of progressive exercises. These are carefully selected to strengthen your body, improve flexibility, and support spinal health. The exercises are introduced gradually, allowing your body to adapt and build resilience over time. It's important to listen to your body, adjusting the intensity and complexity of exercises as needed. This approach ensures that you're not overwhelmed, reducing the risk of injury and promoting steady improvement. Think of it as climbing the mountain step by step, each exercise bringing you closer to the summit of a pain-free existence.

The importance of individualized plans cannot be overstated. Each person's journey to recovery is different, influenced by factors such as age, fitness level, and specific pain triggers. Customizing your recovery plan means considering these variables and tailoring your exercises and activities accordingly. For instance, a young athlete may focus on dynamic stretches and high-intensity workouts, while someone recovering from a sedentary lifestyle might prioritize gentle stretching and core strengthening. This personalized approach maximizes the effectiveness of your recovery efforts, ensuring that they align with your goals and capabilities.

Rest and recovery periods are integral components of any recovery plan. Just as a mountain climber must pause to rest and acclimate, your body requires time to recover and heal. Scheduled rest days allow your muscles to repair and grow stronger, preventing burnout and overuse injuries. Active recovery activities, such as light walking or yoga, can also be beneficial, promoting circulation and maintaining mobility without placing additional stress on your body. These periods of rest are not a sign of weakness but a strategic part of your journey, ensuring that you have the energy and strength needed to continue progressing.

Professional resources play a vital role in supporting your recovery. Consulting with a physical therapist provides expert guidance and tailored exercises that address your specific needs. These professionals can help refine your technique, offering adjustments and recommendations that enhance your recovery experience.

Similarly, seeking chiropractic advice can be invaluable, particularly for issues related to spinal alignment and nerve pressure. Chiropractors offer non-surgical solutions that complement your recovery plan, providing relief and improving overall function. Chiropractors specializing in not only adjustments but exercise recovery include:

American Chiropractic Board of Sports Physicians™:
https://www.acbsp.com/directory/
Diplomate American Chiropractic Rehabilitation Board:
https://acrb.org/location/

Utilizing these resources ensures that you have the support and expertise needed to navigate the complexities of recovery successfully.

Interactive Element: Personal Recovery Planner

Developing a personalized recovery plan can streamline your journey and enhance your outcomes. Use this framework to create a plan that suits your needs:

- **Assessment Phase**: Conduct a self-assessment to understand your pain triggers and physical limitations.

Consider seeking professional evaluations for a comprehensive understanding.

- **Exercise Introduction**: Gradually incorporate exercises that strengthen and stabilize your spine, adjusting intensity based on your progress.
- **Individualization**: Tailor your plan to your unique needs, factoring in fitness level and specific pain conditions.
- **Rest and Recovery**: Schedule regular rest days and engage in active recovery activities to support healing.
- **Professional Consultation**: Utilize healthcare professionals for expert guidance and support.

5.1 SETTING ACHIEVABLE GOALS: SHORT-TERM WINS

Imagine setting off on a road trip without a map or destination. The allure of the open road might seem exciting, but without a clear path, you could end up lost. The same principle applies to recovery from back pain. Establishing realistic goals provides direction and purpose, transforming abstract aspirations into tangible milestones. This is where the SMART goals framework becomes invaluable, guiding you to set goals that are Specific, Measurable, Achievable, Relevant, and Time-bound. By focusing on these criteria, each goal becomes a stepping stone, offering clear indicators of progress and success. For example, a goal like "increase flexibility" becomes "increase hamstring flexibility by 10% within three weeks." This precision not only facilitates tracking but also enhances motivation, as progress becomes visible and concrete.

Consider the power of short-term objectives in your recovery journey. These manageable goals, such as completing a daily stretching routine or achieving a measurable increase in flexibility, provide immediate targets to aim for. They serve as the rungs of a ladder, enabling you to climb steadily toward your broader objectives. Completing a daily stretching routine, for instance, fosters consistency, ingraining positive habits that contribute to long-term recovery. Similarly, measuring an increase in flexibility, whether through improved range of motion or reduced pain during certain movements, offers immediate feedback, validating your efforts and encouraging continued dedication. These small victories accumulate, building momentum and reinforcing your commitment to the recovery process.

Achieving these short-term goals yields profound psychological benefits. Each accomplishment, no matter how small, boosts self-efficacy, the belief in your ability to succeed. This confidence is crucial, propelling you forward even when faced with setbacks or challenges. As you meet and surpass each goal, your commitment to the recovery process strengthens, transforming hope into certainty. The sense of accomplishment derived from these successes fosters a positive mindset, essential for navigating the ups and downs of recovery. Over time, this growing confidence becomes a cornerstone of your approach, empowering you to tackle more ambitious goals with assurance and determination.

Tracking your progress is an integral aspect of goal setting, offering insights into your recovery journey and guiding necessary adjustments. Goal-setting worksheets provide a structured way to document objectives, track achievements, and reflect on experiences. By regularly reviewing these worksheets, you gain a clear understanding of your progression, identifying patterns and areas needing attention. This process fosters accountability, ensuring that you remain focused and motivated. Additionally, these reviews serve as opportunities for celebration, acknowledging the hard work and dedication that have brought you this far. Regular goal reviews highlight your achievements and inform your next steps, ensuring that your recovery remains dynamic and responsive to your evolving needs.

5.2 TRACKING PROGRESS: TOOLS AND TECHNIQUES

In the pursuit of recovery, tracking progress becomes a crucial ally. Imagine navigating an unfamiliar city without a map—tracking is your GPS, guiding you, highlighting areas that need attention, and celebrating milestones reached. Regular monitoring keeps you motivated and provides a tangible sense of achievement. It allows you to see how far you've come, even when daily changes seem imperceptible. By identifying trends and patterns, you can adapt your approach, ensuring continuous improvement and preventing setbacks. This ongoing feedback loop is essential for maintaining momentum and staying on course.

Several tools can assist in this tracking process, each offering unique benefits. Fitness tracking apps like MyFitnessPal provide a user-friendly interface to log exercises, monitor progress, and even track nutrition. They offer detailed insights into your habits and activities, making it easier to spot progress and adjust plans as necessary. For those who prefer a more personal touch, bullet journals serve as an excellent way to record daily experiences, reflections, and achievements. These journals allow for creative freedom, letting you document your journey in a way that resonates with you. By writing down your thoughts and observations, you gain a more profound understanding of your progress, fostering a sense of ownership and commitment.

Metrics are the backbone of effective progress tracking, offering concrete data to evaluate your recovery. Range of motion measurements are invaluable in assessing flexibility and joint health. By regularly measuring how far you can bend or stretch, you gain a clear picture of improvements or areas that need more focus. Pain level assessments also provide critical insights. Using a simple scale from one to ten, you can track how pain fluctuates in response to activities or treatments. This data not only informs your current strategy but also helps in refining plans. Together, these metrics create a comprehensive view of your recovery, empowering you to make informed decisions about your health.

Accountability adds another layer of depth to your progress tracking. Sharing your achievements and challenges with a support group can enhance motivation and provide encouragement. Whether it's a local meet-up or an online forum, these communities offer a space to connect, share experiences, and learn from others. Additionally, partnering with a recovery buddy can be incredibly motivating. This partnership creates a shared commitment, where each person supports and holds the other accountable. The simple act of checking in with someone else can reignite motivation, turning solo efforts into a shared victory. With each tracked step, you move closer to your goals and strengthen the bonds with those supporting your journey.

5.3 ADAPTING YOUR PLAN: HOW TO ADJUST FOR BETTER RESULTS

As you navigate your recovery, adaptability becomes your greatest ally. Recovery is rarely a straight path, and being flexible in your approach is crucial. One key aspect of this adaptability is recognizing when you've hit a plateau. These are moments when progress stalls, and it might feel like you're treading water instead of moving forward. It's important to see these plateaus not as failures, but as signals that your body might need a change in routine or intensity. New pain symptoms may also arise, indicating that certain exercises or activities might be too demanding or need modification. Listening to your body's signals ensures that you respond appropriately, preventing further strain or injury.

When it comes to making informed adjustments, consider incorporating new exercises into your routine. Introducing variety can stimulate muscles in different ways, breaking the monotony and reigniting progress. If you're accustomed to high-impact activities, try integrating low-impact exercises like swimming or cycling that offer similar benefits while being gentler on your joints. On the flip side, during flare-ups or when pain intensifies, it's wise to reduce the intensity of your workouts. This doesn't mean halting all activity but rather scaling back to allow your body to recover. Gentle stretching or light walking can maintain mobility without exacerbating pain. By balancing new challenges with restful activities, you create a harmonious recovery plan that evolves with you.

Regular self-assessment is another cornerstone of an adaptable recovery plan. This involves setting aside time each week to evaluate your progress and the effectiveness of your current approach. A self-evaluation checklist can be a helpful tool in this process, prompting you to consider factors such as pain levels, flexibility improvements, and overall well-being. Reflecting on these aspects offers insights into what's working and what might need tweaking. It empowers you to make proactive changes, ensuring that your recovery plan remains aligned with your goals and physical condition. By engaging in this introspective practice, you cultivate a deeper understanding of your body's needs, enabling you to respond with confidence and precision.

Despite your best efforts, there may be times when professional input is invaluable. Consulting with experts can provide fresh perspectives and tailored modifications to your recovery plan. Physical therapists, for example, can assess your progress and suggest exercises that target specific areas needing improvement.

Their expertise can refine your technique, ensuring that you're maximizing the benefits of each movement. Similarly, chiropractors offer insights into spinal health, addressing alignment issues that might hinder recovery. Their interventions can alleviate discomfort and enhance mobility, complementing your self-directed efforts. Seeking professional guidance doesn't negate your achievements; it enriches your journey, offering support when it's needed most.

5.4 OVERCOMING PLATEAUS: STRATEGIES FOR CONTINUED IMPROVEMENT

In the midst of recovery, you might find yourself at a standstill, a plateau where progress seems to halt. This stagnation can be both frustrating and disheartening, yet it is a common phase in the healing process. Often, repetitive exercise routines contribute to this stagnation. When the body becomes too accustomed to a particular set of movements, the exercises lose their effectiveness, similar to how a musician might plateau if they only practice the same scales. Lack of variety in activities can also play a significant role. Engaging in the same routines day after day doesn't challenge your body in new ways, leading to diminished returns. Recognizing these signs is the first step in overcoming them, allowing you to adjust your approach and reignite progress.

To break through a plateau, one effective strategy is to introduce cross-training activities. Cross-training involves incorporating different forms of exercise that complement your primary routine. For example, if your recovery has focused heavily on strength training, adding cardiovascular activities like swimming or cycling can provide a fresh stimulus for your body. These activities enhance overall fitness and target different muscle groups, reducing the risk of overuse injuries. Another approach is to increase the intensity or duration of your workouts. Gradually adding more weight, extending your exercise time, or intensifying your sessions with interval training can push your limits and spark new progress. Exploring new recovery techniques or therapies, such as massage or acupuncture, can also offer fresh perspectives and benefits, helping your body respond in new and positive ways.

Patience and persistence are key to overcoming plateaus. It's natural to feel impatient when progress slows, but remember that recovery is a marathon, not a sprint. Setting realistic expectations helps maintain focus and motivation. Understand that some days will be better than others, and setbacks are part of the process. Consistency, rather than perfection, is what ultimately leads to success. Embrace each small victory and recognize that persistence often means the difference between stagnation and progress.

Motivational stories can serve as powerful reminders of what's possible. Consider the tale of an amateur marathon runner who faced a plateau after an injury. Despite the frustration, she diversified her training with yoga and strength exercises, eventually breaking through the barrier. Her persistence paid off, leading to improved performance and a newfound passion for whole-body wellness. Or think of an office worker, previously plagued by back pain, who overcame his plateau by incorporating daily walks and adopting a standing desk. These stories are not just about physical transformation but highlight the resilience and adaptability of the human spirit. They remind us that while plateaus are challenging, they are also opportunities for growth and innovation.

By embracing variety, increasing intensity, and maintaining patience, you pave the way for continued improvement. The process may be slow, but each step forward is a testament to your commitment and strength.

5.5 CELEBRATING SUCCESSES: MOTIVATION FOR THE LONG HAUL

Recovery can often feel like a long, winding road, marked by ups and downs. Embracing each achievement along the way can transform this journey into an inspiring experience. Celebrating milestones is not just about acknowledging progress; it's about infusing energy and enthusiasm into your recovery. Imagine the satisfaction of reaching a personal best in flexibility or achieving a new strength goal. These moments are worth celebrating, as they signify hard work and perseverance paying off. Recognizing these achievements serves as a powerful reminder of your capabilities, reinforcing your motivation to keep pushing forward. Each milestone celebrated is a testament to your dedication, an opportunity to pause and appreciate how far you've come. This recognition is not only rewarding, but essential for maintaining momentum, as it fuels your desire to continue thriving in your recovery process.

Finding meaningful ways to reward yourself can add a layer of joy to your accomplishments. Consider treating yourself to a massage, which serves as a delightful indulgence and offers therapeutic benefits for your muscles and mind. Alternatively, engaging in a favorite activity without pain serves as its own celebration. Whether it's a leisurely hike, a dance class, or simply playing with your kids, experiencing these moments pain-free is a triumph worth savoring. These rewards are not just about indulgence; they're about acknowledging the hard work you've put in and the progress you've made. By choosing rewards that resonate with you personally, you create an incentive that is both meaningful and motivating, encouraging continued effort and dedication.

The act of celebrating successes has profound psychological benefits, reinforcing positive behavior and boosting self-image. When you take the time to acknowledge what you've achieved, you validate your efforts and build confidence in your abilities. This enhanced self-image can have a ripple effect, influencing other aspects of your life. Confidence gained through recovery achievements can translate into improved performance in your work, sports, and daily interactions. It becomes a cycle of positivity, where each success fuels further success, creating a momentum that propels you forward. This cycle is integral to sustaining motivation, as it transforms challenges into opportunities for growth, encouraging you to tackle each new goal with renewed vigor.

Cultivating a mindset of continuous improvement is key to long-term success. View each milestone not as a finish line, but as a stepping stone towards ongoing progress and lifelong health. After achieving a goal, take a moment to reflect on your personal growth and the journey that brought you here. This reflection not only provides insight into your progress but also highlights the resilience and determination you've developed along the way. Use these reflections as a springboard for setting new goals, challenging yourself to reach even greater heights. This mindset fosters an attitude of lifelong learning and improvement, ensuring that your recovery journey continues to evolve and adapt as you do. By embracing this perspective, you maintain motivation and enrich your life with a sense of purpose and achievement.

6

THE MIND-BODY CONNECTION

Imagine standing on a tightrope, balancing precariously while the world watches. This delicate equilibrium mirrors the relationship between mind and body, especially when back pain enters the scene. Stress, often an unseen adversary, intensifies this struggle, manifesting its effects through physiological and psychological pathways. When stress takes hold, it seizes the muscles, inducing tension that wraps around your spine like an unyielding grip. This stress-induced muscle tension is not just a fleeting discomfort; it can amplify existing pain, transforming minor aches into relentless throbs.

The body's response to stress involves more than just physical tension. Deep within, a cascade of hormonal changes takes place, affecting how pain is perceived. The adrenal glands release cortisol, a hormone that, while essential for managing acute stress, can exacerbate pain when levels remain elevated over time. This hormonal response can alter your perception of pain, making sensations feel more intense and harder to ignore. The interplay between stress and the body highlights how intricately connected our mental and physical states are, and understanding this can be key to managing back pain effectively.

Identifying the sources of stress in your life is the first step toward alleviating its impact on your back. Work-related stress is a common culprit, with tight deadlines, long hours, and high expectations creating a pressure cooker environment. This stress doesn't evaporate when you leave the office; it follows you home, intertwining with personal relationship challenges. Whether it's disagreements with loved ones or the strain of maintaining connections, these emotional stressors can weigh heavily on your back, literally and figuratively. Recognizing these stressors is crucial, as it allows you to address them directly and reduce their grip on your well-being.

The relationship between stress and pain is cyclical, forming a negative feedback loop that's difficult to escape. Pain increases stress levels, as you worry about its implications on your health and daily life. This heightened stress, in turn, exacerbates the pain, creating a vicious cycle that's both physically and emotionally draining. Breaking free from this cycle requires a proactive approach. It's about taking steps to manage stress effectively, thereby reducing its influence on your pain levels. By addressing the root of the stress, you can alleviate the symptoms and gain a sense of control over your body.

Practical techniques for stress reduction can provide relief and empower you to manage back pain more effectively. Deep breathing exercises are a simple yet powerful tool. By focusing on slow, deliberate breaths, you activate the body's relaxation response, reducing stress-induced muscle tension and promoting a sense of calm. Progressive muscle relaxation is another technique that involves tensing and then relaxing each muscle group, helping you become more aware of physical tension and how to release it. These methods, while seemingly small, can have a profound impact on your stress levels and, by extension, your back pain.

Interactive Element: Stress Reduction Exercise

Try this simple deep breathing exercise:

1. Sit comfortably with your back straight. Close your eyes and place one hand on your chest and the other on your abdomen.
2. Breathe in slowly through your nose, feeling your abdomen rise as it fills with air.
3. Hold your breath for a moment, then exhale slowly through your mouth.
4. Focus on the sensation of your breath, repeating this cycle for five minutes.

Incorporating these exercises into your daily routine can create a buffer against stress, helping to prevent it from spiraling into pain. By taking control of your stress response, you can foster resilience and promote a healthier, more balanced life. Remember, the mind and body are not separate entities; they are intertwined, and nurturing one can lead to healing in the other.

6.1 MINDFULNESS AND MEDITATION: TOOLS FOR PAIN MANAGEMENT

Mindfulness is more than a buzzword; it's a tool that can transform how you perceive and manage pain. At its core, mindfulness is about cultivating present-moment awareness—being fully engaged with your current experience without judgment. This practice encourages you to acknowledge pain without labeling it as good or bad, simply observing it as it is. By fostering acceptance of physical sensations, mindfulness helps reduce the emotional turmoil that often accompanies chronic pain. Imagine sitting quietly, focusing on your breath, and noticing sensations in your body without the urge to change them. This approach can diminish the cycle of tension and stress, making pain more manageable.

Meditation offers a structured way to practice mindfulness, with various techniques tailored to different needs. Guided imagery meditation invites you to picture serene scenes, like a tranquil beach or a peaceful forest, directing your attention away from discomfort and reducing pain intensity. In contrast, loving-kindness meditation involves silently repeating phrases that cultivate compassion towards yourself and others. This practice can soften the grip of pain by fostering a sense of connection and empathy. Both methods promote relaxation and emotional balance, crucial elements in managing back pain effectively. Regular meditation practice can be a game-changer, offering a respite from the relentless nature of chronic discomfort.

The benefits of consistent mindfulness and meditation practice extend beyond immediate relief. Over time, you'll likely notice a reduction in pain intensity and an improvement in emotional regulation. As mindfulness strengthens your awareness, you become more adept at recognizing tension and addressing it before it escalates. This heightened awareness can prevent pain from dominating your thoughts and emotions, creating space for other aspects of life. Additionally, meditation encourages a shift in how you relate to pain, reducing its emotional impact. With persistence, these practices can lead to profound changes in how you experience pain, enhancing your overall quality of life.

Starting a meditation routine doesn't require a significant time commitment or elaborate setup. Begin by creating a meditation space, a quiet corner of your home where you feel comfortable and undisturbed. This dedicated area can help signal to your mind that it's time to relax and focus inward. Once your space is ready, commit to a simple five-minute daily mindfulness practice. Sit or lie down in a comfortable position, close your eyes, and bring your attention to your breath. Notice the rise and fall of your chest, the sensation of air flowing in and out. When your mind wanders, gently guide it back to your breath without judgment. This practice, though brief, can have a cumulative effect, gradually increasing your capacity for mindfulness and pain awareness.

Reflection Section: Creating Your Meditation Space

Think about what makes you feel calm and centered. Is it a particular scent, like lavender or sandalwood? Perhaps soft lighting or a specific chair that supports your posture. Gather these elements to create a meditation space that invites relaxation and focus. Reflect on how this space makes you feel and how you can adjust it to enhance your practice. As you engage with mindfulness and meditation, remember that it's a personal journey—tailor it to fit your unique needs and preferences.

6.2 COGNITIVE BEHAVIORAL STRATEGIES FOR CHRONIC PAIN

Cognitive Behavioral Therapy (CBT) emerges as a cornerstone in managing chronic pain by reshaping the thought patterns that often exacerbate our physical discomfort. At its core, CBT is about understanding that our thoughts, feelings, and behaviors are interconnected. By altering one, we can influence the others. In the realm of pain management, this means identifying and challenging the cognitive distortions that can lead to increased pain perception. Cognitive restructuring, one of CBT's key components, involves recognizing these distorted thoughts and replacing them with more balanced, realistic ones. For instance, if you catch yourself thinking, "I'll never get better," CBT encourages you to challenge this belief and consider a more positive perspective, such as, "I am making progress, and I have tools to manage my pain."

Behavioral activation is another vital aspect, focusing on engaging in activities that promote a sense of accomplishment and joy. Chronic pain often leads to a cycle of avoidance, where you may stop doing things you love for fear of worsening the pain. Behavioral activation breaks this cycle by encouraging you to gradually reintroduce these activities, providing positive reinforcement and enhancing your quality of life. This strategic approach to behavior can significantly shift your focus away from pain and towards the moments that bring you happiness and fulfillment.

Recognizing cognitive distortions is crucial in this process. These distortions can magnify pain and diminish hope. Catastrophizing, for example, involves imagining the worst-case scenario, often leading to increased anxiety and pain perception. It's the voice in your head that whispers, "This pain will ruin everything." Overgeneralization, another distortion, involves taking a single negative event and applying it broadly, such as believing that one bad day means every day will be painful. Challenging these thoughts is key. When you notice these patterns, pause and question their validity. Ask yourself, "Is this thought based on facts, or is it an emotional reaction?" This self-reflection can diffuse the emotional charge and help you see the situation more clearly.

Practical techniques from CBT offer actionable strategies for managing chronic pain. Thought records are an effective tool, encouraging you to document your thoughts, feelings, and behaviors in response to pain. This practice helps you identify patterns and triggers, providing insights into how your thoughts influence your experience of pain. By writing down these reflections, you gain a new perspective, often realizing that some of your beliefs about pain might not hold up under scrutiny. Another CBT strategy involves scheduling pleasant activities, deliberately setting aside time for things that bring you joy. Whether it's a hobby, spending time with loved ones, or simply enjoying a good book, these activities can elevate your mood and reduce the focus on pain.

Sometimes, professional guidance is beneficial, especially if chronic pain significantly impacts your daily life. Indicators that might suggest seeking a therapist trained in CBT include persistent negative thoughts about pain, difficulty engaging in daily activities, or a sense of hopelessness about managing pain. A therapist can provide tailored strategies, offering support and expertise to guide you through the process. They help you set realistic goals and offer accountability, ensuring you stay on track. Additionally, they can teach you more advanced techniques, deepening your understanding of how to navigate the complexities of chronic pain. Engaging with a professional can provide clarity and direction, empowering you to regain control over your pain and life.

Cognitive Behavioral Therapy offers a structured, evidence-based approach to managing chronic pain. By altering how you think about and respond to pain, CBT equips you with the tools to reduce its impact on your life. It's about shifting the narrative from one of helplessness to one of empowerment, where you actively participate in your healing process.

6.3 EMOTIONAL RESILIENCE: BUILDING A STRONGER YOU

Emotional resilience is the ability to adapt and thrive despite life's challenges, including the persistent discomfort of back pain. It's about cultivating the strength to face adversity with a positive outlook. This kind of resilience isn't just about enduring hardship; it's about growing stronger through it. When you build emotional resilience, you enhance your ability to cope with pain and the stress that often accompanies it. Imagine it as a buffer, absorbing the shocks of life's difficulties and allowing you to maintain balance. This adaptability in the face of stress allows you to navigate pain's ups and downs without losing hope or motivation. By focusing on maintaining a positive outlook, you shift your perspective, viewing setbacks as opportunities for growth rather than insurmountable obstacles.

Building emotional resilience involves several key strategies. Developing a support network is a crucial component. Having people you can rely on, whether friends, family, or support groups, provides a sense of belonging and understanding. They offer a shoulder to lean on during tough times and celebrate with you during victories. This network acts as a safety net, catching you when you're at your lowest and lifting you higher. Another powerful tool in your resilience-building arsenal is practicing gratitude. By acknowledging the positive aspects of your life, no matter how small, you foster a mindset of abundance and appreciation. This practice shifts focus from what is lacking to what is present, nurturing a more optimistic outlook.

The role of self-compassion in fostering resilience cannot be overstated. Being kind to yourself, especially when faced with challenges, is vital. Self-compassion involves treating yourself with the same kindness and understanding you would offer a friend in distress. It's about recognizing that everyone struggles and that it's okay to have moments of weakness. Embracing self-compassion exercises, such as writing yourself a letter of encouragement or taking time for self-care, reinforces this mindset. These exercises help you build a foundation of self-kindness, which strengthens your resilience. By accepting your imperfections and forgiving your missteps, you create an inner environment that supports healing and growth.

Consider the story of a chronic pain survivor who embodies emotional resilience. After years of enduring relentless back pain, she decided to change her narrative. Instead of focusing on her limitations, she chose to celebrate her small victories, like walking a bit longer each day. She surrounded herself with a supportive community, sharing her journey and learning from others. Her practice of gratitude became a daily ritual, shifting her focus to the beauty in her life. Through self-compassion, she forgave herself for days when pain held her back and celebrated those when she triumphed. Her story illustrates how resilience is not about eliminating pain, but about thriving despite it.

By adopting these strategies, you can cultivate emotional resilience and transform your relationship with pain. It's about developing a mindset that embraces challenges as opportunities for growth, supported by a network of allies and a foundation of self-kindness. Emotional resilience doesn't eliminate pain, but it empowers you to rise above it, growing stronger with each step forward.

6.4 THE POWER OF POSITIVE THINKING IN RECOVERY

In the realm of recovery, the mindset you adopt can be as influential as the physical treatments you pursue. Positive thinking is not merely wishful thinking; it is a powerful force that can profoundly affect your healing process. At its core, a positive outlook shifts your focus from limitations to possibilities, fostering an environment where recovery can thrive. This optimism acts as a catalyst, enhancing your body's natural healing abilities. When you approach your recovery with hope and determination, you create a mental landscape that encourages progress and resilience. The psychological benefits of maintaining a positive mindset are well-documented, with studies showing that individuals who cultivate optimism often experience faster recovery times and improved outcomes. This is because positive thinking reduces stress and anxiety, which are known to impede healing. By viewing your recovery journey through a lens of positivity, you empower yourself to overcome obstacles and embrace each small victory along the way.

To cultivate a positive mindset, consider integrating techniques that reinforce optimism into your daily routine. Affirmations, for instance, are simple yet effective tools for reinforcing positive beliefs. By repeating affirmations such as "I am strong and capable of healing," you program your mind to focus on your strengths and potential. Visualization exercises can also be transformative. Picture yourself engaging in activities that currently seem challenging or unattainable. Feel the joy and satisfaction of achieving these goals, and let this mental rehearsal guide your actions. Journaling positive experiences is another powerful method for fostering positivity. Each day, take a moment to reflect on and write down three things you are grateful for or proud of. This practice shifts your attention from what might be going wrong to what is going right, reinforcing a sense of achievement and gratitude.

Maintaining a positive mindset is not without its challenges. Setbacks are inevitable, and when they occur, it's easy to slip into negative thought patterns. Recognizing these thoughts is the first step to overcoming them. When you find yourself dwelling on a setback, challenge its validity. Ask yourself if this obstacle truly defines your recovery journey, or if it's simply a temporary detour. By reframing setbacks as opportunities for growth, you can maintain your momentum and continue moving forward. Identifying negative thought patterns, such as self-doubt or fear of failure, is also crucial. Once you recognize these thoughts, replace them with affirmations that reinforce your determination and resilience.

Creating a supportive environment plays a vital role in sustaining positivity throughout your recovery. Surround yourself with people who uplift and encourage you. Whether it's family, friends, or support groups, having a network of positive influences can provide the encouragement and motivation you need. Establishing a positive daily routine is equally important. Incorporate activities that bring you joy and relaxation, such as listening to music, spending time in nature, or engaging in creative pursuits. A structured routine that prioritizes self-care and positivity can enhance your overall well-being and support your recovery.

6.5 YOGA FOR THE MIND AND BODY: A COMPREHENSIVE GUIDE

Yoga stands as a bridge between the physical and mental realms, offering dual benefits that enhance both flexibility and well-being. This practice, rooted in ancient traditions, is much more than physical postures; it's a holistic approach to health. On the physical side, yoga strengthens muscles, improves balance, and increases range of motion. For those with back pain, these aspects are crucial. Stretching and strengthening the muscles around the spine can alleviate discomfort and prevent future issues. Meanwhile, the mental benefits are equally significant. Yoga encourages a state of calm and focus, effectively reducing stress and its harmful effects on the body. As you move through poses, your mind focuses on breath and form, fostering a sense of peace that can be elusive in our fast-paced world.

For those seeking relief from lower back pain, specific yoga poses offer targeted benefits. Child's Pose, for instance, is a gentle stretch that relaxes the lower back and hips. By kneeling and extending your arms forward on the floor, you encourage your back to release tension. The Cat-Cow Stretch is another effective movement, promoting flexibility in the spine. As you alternate between arching and rounding your back, this dynamic flow massages your spine, enhancing mobility. Downward-Facing Dog, a staple in many yoga routines, stretches the entire back body, from the shoulders to the hamstrings. This pose not only lengthens the spine but also strengthens the arms and legs, contributing to overall stability. These poses create a foundation for a more flexible, resilient back, offering relief from pain and fostering long-term health.

Starting a yoga practice doesn't require much more than a willingness to explore. Whether at home or in a class setting, there are many ways to begin. Choosing a yoga style that suits your needs and preferences is the first step. Hatha yoga, known for its gentle pace, is excellent for beginners or those with physical limitations. Vinyasa yoga offers a more dynamic flow, perfect for those who enjoy a bit of challenge. Setting realistic goals is crucial; begin with short sessions and gradually increase the time as you become more comfortable. Consistency is key, so finding a routine that fits your schedule will help you maintain the practice. Experimenting with different styles and instructors can also enrich your experience, allowing you to find what resonates best.

Adapting yoga to individual needs ensures accessibility for everyone, regardless of ability level. Props like blocks and straps can modify poses, making them more approachable. For instance, a block under the hands in Downward-Facing Dog can reduce strain on the wrists and shoulders. Straps can assist in poses requiring flexibility, such as seated forward bends, allowing you to reach comfortably while maintaining proper alignment. Modifying poses for limited mobility might involve using a chair for support or practicing against a wall. These adjustments ensure that yoga remains inclusive, providing benefits to all who practice. Listening to your body and respecting its limits is vital, ensuring that each session is both challenging and nurturing.

As you integrate yoga into your life, you may find it transforms your approach to both movement and stillness. The practice cultivates awareness, helping you tune into your body's signals and respond with care. It encourages a balance between effort and ease, mirroring the balance needed in daily life. Yoga is not just an exercise; it's a way to connect with yourself, fostering a sense of harmony and peace that extends beyond the mat. Whether you're seeking physical relief or a mental reset, yoga offers a path to both, enhancing your quality of life in subtle yet profound ways.

7

PREVENTIVE MEASURES FOR ACTIVE LIFESTYLES

Imagine standing at the starting line of a race, the thrill of anticipation coursing through your veins. You know that every second counts and that precision in movement is key to reaching the finish line without faltering. The same principle applies to injury prevention in physical activities. Proper technique is not just about enhancing performance; it is a crucial safeguard against injuries that could sideline you from your favorite activities. Whether you are lifting weights, running, or practicing yoga, the foundation of injury prevention lies in mastering the correct form, ensuring that your body operates in harmony with its natural mechanics.

The importance of proper technique cannot be overstated. It serves as the bedrock of safe and effective physical activity. Correct alignment and posture are vital components, ensuring that your movements are fluid and efficient. When your body is aligned correctly, the stress on muscles and joints is minimized, reducing the risk of strain and injury. Controlled breathing techniques further enhance your performance, allowing for better oxygen flow and concentration. This focus on form is not just for athletes; it benefits anyone engaged in physical activity. By prioritizing technique, you optimize performance and safeguard against the pitfalls of injury.

Maintaining proper form across various activities requires attention to detail and mindfulness. Engaging your core during exercises is a fundamental tip, as it provides stability and support to your spine. A strong core acts like a natural brace, helping you maintain balance and control. Keeping the spine neutral during lifts, such as deadlifts, is another crucial guideline. A neutral spine ensures that the weight is distributed evenly, preventing undue stress on any single segment. This alignment protects the vertebrae and surrounding muscles, reducing the chance of injury. By consistently applying these principles, you create a solid foundation for safe and effective exercise.

However, even with the best intentions, common technique errors can lead to injury. One frequent mistake is rounding the back during deadlifts, which places excessive strain on the lower back and increases the risk of injury. Similarly, overextending in yoga poses can compromise joint integrity and lead to strains. Recognizing these errors is the first step in correcting them. By being aware of potential pitfalls, you can consciously adjust your form, ensuring that each movement is executed safely. This awareness is crucial for long-term health and well-being, allowing you to enjoy physical activities without the threat of injury.

Seeking professional instruction is an invaluable investment in your health and performance. Coaches and trainers provide expert guidance, ensuring that your technique is precise and effective. One-on-one coaching sessions offer personalized feedback and tailored exercises that address your specific needs. These sessions allow for real-time adjustments, helping you refine your form and avoid common mistakes. Video analysis is another powerful tool, offering visual feedback that highlights areas for improvement. By reviewing footage of your movements, you gain a deeper understanding of your technique, enabling you to make informed adjustments. This professional insight is a key component of injury prevention, providing the knowledge and support needed to thrive in your chosen activities.

Interactive Element: Video Analysis Checklist

Developing a checklist for video analysis can streamline your efforts and enhance your performance. Use this framework to evaluate your technique:

- **Camera Setup**: Ensure your camera captures a full view of the exercise, focusing on key angles.
- **Body Alignment**: Check that your spine, hips, and limbs maintain correct alignment throughout the movement.
- **Core Engagement**: Observe whether your core remains activated, providing stability and support.
- **Breathing Patterns**: Note your breathing technique, ensuring it is controlled and synchronized with your movements.
- **Error Identification**: Identify any rounding, overextending, or misalignments to address and correct.

By prioritizing proper technique and seeking professional guidance, you lay the groundwork for a safe and successful journey in physical activities. This commitment to form enhances performance and protects your body, allowing you to pursue your passions with confidence and resilience.

7.1 WARM-UP ROUTINES: PREPARING YOUR BODY FOR ACTIVITY

Imagine getting ready to run. Your muscles are cold, your joints stiff, and your body feels sluggish. Now, picture how a few minutes of warming up can change that. Warm-ups aren't just a prelude to exercise; they are a crucial element that primes your body for the demands ahead. As you elevate your heart rate, blood flow increases, delivering oxygen and nutrients to your muscles. This process enhances muscle elasticity, making them more pliable and less prone to strains. Joints become more flexible, moving more freely and reducing the risk of wear and tear. The benefits are clear: a well-prepared body performs better and with a reduced risk of injury.

Dynamic warm-up exercises offer an ideal way to prepare your body for activity. Unlike static stretches, which are best saved for after your workout, dynamic movements use muscle force and momentum to increase your range of motion. Picture yourself doing arm circles, feeling the gentle stretch across your shoulders, or performing leg swings to loosen up your hips. High knees and butt kicks further elevate your heart rate, engaging your legs and core. These movements aren't just about flexibility; they activate the muscles you'll use during your workout, ensuring they are ready for action. By incorporating these exercises, you set the stage for a more effective and enjoyable session.

Tailoring your warm-up to your specific sport can make all the difference. For basketball players, dribbling drills not only warm up the legs but also refine hand-eye coordination. These drills simulate game conditions, preparing both mind and body. Martial artists might engage in shadow-boxing, a practice that combines footwork, punches, and defensive moves. This exercise not only warms up the body but also sharpens focus and technique. By aligning your warm-up with your activity, you ensure that the muscles and skills needed are honed and ready, reducing the chance of injury and enhancing performance.

Starting slow and building intensity is a wise approach to warming up. Think of it as gently waking up your body, allowing it to transition from rest to full activity. Progressive tempo runs, where you gradually increase your pace, are an excellent example. They prepare your cardiovascular system and muscles for the demands of a more intense workout. Similarly, in strength training, begin with lighter weights and gradually increase the resistance. This gradual build-up allows your muscles and joints to adapt, minimizing the risk of strain. Emphasizing gradual intensity helps prevent injury and maximizes the efficiency of your workout, setting the tone for success.

7.2 RECOVERY PRACTICES: ESSENTIAL POST-ACTIVITY RITUALS

After a demanding workout or intense sports session, your body needs time to recalibrate. Post-activity recovery isn't just an afterthought; it's a critical component of your exercise regimen. Engaging in effective recovery practices helps your muscles repair, reduces soreness, and prepares you for your next bout of activity. One key aspect is the cooldown phase, which transitions your body from high energy to rest. Cooldown stretches are paramount in this phase. They help elongate muscle fibers that have contracted during exercise, preventing stiffness and maintaining flexibility. By gradually slowing your heart rate and breathing, cooldown stretches signal to your body that it's time to shift gears, facilitating a smoother recovery process.

Hydration is another cornerstone of recovery. When you exercise, your body loses fluids through sweat, which can lead to dehydration if not replenished. Drinking water post-activity is vital, but adding electrolyte drinks to your regimen can further enhance recovery. Electrolytes, such as sodium and potassium, aid in balancing the body's fluid levels, ensuring that your muscles function optimally. This rehydration process helps replenish the nutrients lost during exercise, reducing the risk of cramps and fatigue. Keeping a water bottle and electrolyte drink handy ensures you can start the rehydration process immediately, optimizing your body's recovery capabilities.

Incorporating effective cooldown exercises can also aid in recovery. Static stretching sequences, where you hold a stretch for a prolonged period, help release tension in the muscles and increase flexibility. These stretches are best performed after the bulk of your activity, targeting major muscle groups like the hamstrings, quads, and shoulders. Gentle yoga flows are another excellent option, combining movement and breath to relax the body and mind. Poses like the child's pose or cat-cow stretch promote relaxation and spinal health, aligning the body and easing muscle tension. These exercises enhance physical recovery and calm the mind, reducing stress and promoting a sense of well-being.

Nutrition plays a pivotal role in muscle recovery and energy replenishment. After exercise, your muscles are primed to absorb nutrients, making it an ideal time to consume a protein-rich snack. Foods like Greek yogurt, nuts, or a protein shake provide the amino acids necessary for muscle repair. Carbohydrates are equally important, as they replenish glycogen stores depleted during physical exertion. A balanced post-activity snack ensures that your body has the resources it needs to recover efficiently and prepare for future challenges. By prioritizing nutrition, you equip your body with the fuel it needs to repair and rebuild, enhancing overall performance.

Rest and sleep are fundamental to full recovery. Your body does much of its repair work while you sleep, making quality rest crucial. Establishing a calming bedtime routine can significantly improve sleep quality. Consider activities like reading, gentle stretching, or listening to soothing music before bed. These practices signal to your body that it's time to wind down, promoting relaxation and deeper sleep. Avoiding screens and caffeine in the evening further enhances your ability to fall asleep and stay asleep. Quality sleep not only supports physical recovery but also boosts mental clarity and mood, preparing you for the next day's activities with renewed energy and focus.

7.3 CROSS-TRAINING: DIVERSIFYING FOR BETTER SPINE HEALTH

Imagine you're an artist, painting a masterpiece. You wouldn't rely on a single color to bring your vision to life, would you? The same principle applies to fitness and spine health. Cross-training is akin to having a palette full of colors, each one contributing to a well-rounded and balanced picture of fitness. It involves engaging in various exercises that target different muscle groups, enhancing overall fitness and reducing the risk of injury. When you incorporate cross-training into your routine, you achieve balanced muscle development. This means that no single group of muscles bears the brunt of your workouts, minimizing the wear and tear that can lead to injury. Additionally, cross-training boosts cardiovascular endurance, as it challenges your heart and lungs in diverse ways, keeping your body agile and responsive.

Consider the benefits of incorporating activities like swimming and Pilates into your fitness routine. Swimming offers a joint-friendly cardio workout, as the buoyancy of the water reduces the impact on your joints while still providing resistance to build strength and stamina. It's a refreshing way to improve cardiovascular health without the stress that high-impact activities like running might impose on your spine. Similarly, Pilates focuses on core strengthening, enhancing the muscles that support your spine and posture. By improving core stability, you protect your back from strains and enhance your ability to perform other exercises safely and effectively. These activities complement your primary sports or workouts and enrich your overall fitness, providing a holistic approach to maintaining a healthy spine.

Cross-training is particularly effective in preventing overuse injuries. Imagine running every single day without a break—it would be like playing the same note repeatedly on a piano. Eventually, the melody would become monotonous, and your body, like the piano, would wear down. By alternating between high-impact and low-impact activities, you allow different muscle groups to recover while keeping your body engaged. This variation reduces the risk of repetitive stress injuries, as it distributes the physical demands across a broader spectrum of activities. For instance, if your primary sport is running, incorporating cycling or swimming into your routine on alternate days provides cardiovascular benefits while giving your legs a break from the pounding impact. This balance is crucial for longevity in any fitness regimen.

To integrate cross-training into your weekly schedule, consider a template that mixes different activities. For example, dedicate one day to running for cardiovascular endurance, followed by a day of cycling to engage different muscles. Include strength training sessions that focus on building muscle and enhancing bone density, providing a well-rounded approach to fitness. On another day, engage in a Pilates class to concentrate on core strength and flexibility. Such a schedule keeps your routine fresh and exciting and ensures that your body remains balanced and well-conditioned. By diversifying your workouts, you cultivate a resilient and adaptable body, ready to tackle any challenge.

Cross-training is not just a buzzword in the fitness world—it's a strategic approach to achieving and maintaining spine health while enhancing overall fitness. By embracing a variety of activities, you improve physical performance and protect your body from the pitfalls of repetitive strain. This innovative approach encourages you to explore new exercises, keeping your routine dynamic and engaging. Whether you're an athlete looking to boost performance or someone seeking a balanced fitness regimen, cross-training offers a pathway to a healthier, more vibrant life.

7.4 INCORPORATING ACTIVE RECOVERY INTO YOUR ROUTINE

Active recovery is a subtle yet powerful concept often overlooked in fitness regimens. Unlike complete rest, which involves taking a full break from physical activities, active recovery keeps the body moving with low-intensity exercises. This approach promotes circulation, helping to deliver oxygen and nutrients to tired muscles, facilitating repair and growth. Imagine it as a gentle walk through a garden rather than a full stop at a traffic light. Activities such as walking or light jogging provide the perfect balance, allowing your body to maintain movement without the strain of intense exercise. Gentle swimming sessions, too, offer a soothing environment where muscles can unwind, buoyed by water that alleviates joint pressure.

The timing of active recovery plays a crucial role in its effectiveness. Consider the day following an intense training session; this is an ideal moment for active recovery. Your muscles, having been pushed to their limits, benefit from gentle movements that prevent stiffness and soreness while still engaging the body. During recovery weeks, when you intentionally dial back the intensity of your exercise routine, active recovery becomes your ally. It helps maintain your fitness level without overtaxing your system, ensuring that you remain on track with your goals while giving your body the respite it needs.

Beyond the physical benefits, active recovery holds significant psychological advantages. Engaging in light activities releases endorphins, those feel-good chemicals that naturally elevate your mood and reduce stress. Picture the calm that washes over you during a leisurely stroll or the sense of freedom you feel as you glide through a pool. These activities not only refresh the body but invigorate the mind, providing mental relaxation through movement that lifts your spirits and clears your thoughts. In a world where stress is a constant companion, the mental reprieve offered by active recovery is invaluable.

Incorporating active recovery into your routine doesn't demand drastic changes. It can be as simple as incorporating a short walk after a workout, or dedicating a day to leisurely cycling. The key is to choose activities that you enjoy and that complement your existing fitness regimen, allowing you to stay active without overexerting yourself. By weaving these gentle exercises into your schedule, you create a balanced approach that supports both physical and mental well-being. Active recovery is about listening to what your body needs and responding with kindness and care, ensuring that fitness remains a sustainable and enjoyable part of your life.

7.5 LISTENING TO YOUR BODY: SIGNS YOU SHOULDN'T IGNORE

Picture this: you're in the middle of a workout, pushing through reps with determination. Suddenly, a sharp pain pierces through your focus, demanding attention. This is your body speaking, and it's crucial to listen. Body awareness is your internal radar, guiding you to recognize when something isn't right. It's about tuning into the subtle signals your body sends, preventing minor issues from escalating into significant injuries. Fatigue and pain are not hurdles to power through; they are warnings that your body needs a break. Ignoring these signals can lead to more than just discomfort—it can result in setbacks that derail your fitness goals.

When it comes to identifying warning signs, certain symptoms should never be brushed aside. Persistent sharp pain is a clear red flag, indicating that something more serious might be at play. It's different from the usual muscle soreness that follows a good workout. This pain is more intense, often localized, and doesn't subside with rest. Swelling and inflammation are also indicators that require immediate attention. They often accompany injuries like sprains or strains, signaling that the body needs time to heal. Catching these signs early and addressing them promptly can prevent further damage and facilitate faster recovery. It's about being proactive, taking steps to care for your body when it whispers for help, rather than waiting until it screams.

Responding to these signs with urgency is crucial. Taking rest days isn't a sign of weakness; it's a strategic move that allows your body to repair and strengthen. Rest gives your muscles time to recover, reducing the risk of overuse injuries. If symptoms persist despite rest, it's wise to consult healthcare professionals. They offer expertise that can diagnose underlying issues, providing guidance on the best course of action. Whether it's a physical therapist offering exercises tailored to your needs or a doctor assessing the extent of an injury, professional advice ensures that you're not navigating recovery blindly. Addressing potential problems early keeps you on track, preventing long-term setbacks and fostering a sustainable fitness journey.

Improving body awareness involves cultivating practices that enhance your ability to listen and interpret bodily signals. Mindful movement exercises are a fantastic starting point. Activities such as yoga or tai chi emphasize slow, deliberate movements that heighten your awareness of how your body feels and moves. These practices encourage you to focus on the present moment, fostering a deeper connection with your physical self. Journaling physical sensations and responses is another effective technique. By documenting how your body feels during and after activities, you create a log that helps identify patterns and triggers. This reflective practice can highlight improvements or recurring issues, offering insights that guide your approach to exercise and recovery.

As you integrate these strategies into your routine, you begin to develop an intuitive understanding of your body's needs. This awareness empowers you to make informed decisions, whether it's pushing harder in a workout or opting for a day of rest. Listening to your body becomes second nature, a practice that prevents injury and enhances overall well-being. By embracing this mindset, you create a foundation for a healthy, active lifestyle that respects and responds to your body's unique signals.

As this chapter concludes, remember that listening to your body is not just a skill but a lifelong practice. It's about finding the balance between pushing limits and nurturing oneself, ensuring that physical activity remains a source of strength and joy. In the next chapter, we'll explore how mental resilience complements physical health, creating a holistic approach to well-being.

8

REAL STORIES AND LONG-TERM SUCCESS

In the quiet moments of reflection, when we consider the struggles and triumphs of our lives, stories emerge as powerful tools of transformation. They offer hope, guidance, and a sense of shared experience. As you navigate through the challenges of back pain, these narratives become beacons of light, illuminating paths you might have thought impassable. The tales of individuals who have walked similar paths and emerged victorious are not just stories; they are testaments to the resilience of the human spirit, providing a glimpse into the profound impact that targeted exercises and lifestyle changes can have on one's life.

Take, for instance, a young athlete named Emma, whose journey epitomizes the challenges and victories that come with overcoming chronic pain. At just 17, Emma was a promising gymnast, her future a tapestry of potential and ambition. Yet, a persistent, gnawing pain in her lower back threatened to unravel her dreams. Initial attempts at traditional treatments offered little reprieve, and frustration mounted as she faced the prospect of sidelining her passion. It was during a particularly disheartening practice, as she struggled to complete a routine, that Emma realized something had to change. She turned to a tailored exercise regimen, guided by evidence-based practices that focused on strengthening her core and improving flexibility. These exercises alleviated her pain and empowered her to regain her confidence. Each day brought new strength and, eventually, a return to the sport she loved.

Then there's David, whose story is a testament to the power of adopting ergonomic practices in a seemingly mundane office environment. As a desk worker, David spent endless hours hunched over a computer, unaware of the toll it took on his back. Persistent discomfort became a constant companion, overshadowing his professional and personal life. The turning point came during a routine visit to his chiropractor, who introduced him to the concept of ergonomics. With a few simple adjustments—an ergonomic chair, a properly positioned monitor, and regular standing breaks—David experienced a transformation. His pain subsided, replaced by a newfound vitality that permeated all aspects of his life. The simple act of aligning his workspace with his body's needs marked a pivotal change, one that underscored the profound connection between our environment and well-being.

Consider also the journey of Margaret, a senior who faced the daunting prospect of losing mobility due to back pain. For Margaret, mornings were once filled with the joy of gardening, a beloved hobby that had become increasingly difficult due to her discomfort. The fear of losing this cherished activity weighed heavily on her. It wasn't until a friend introduced her to gentle exercises that focused on flexibility and core stability that she began to see a shift. Each movement, though small, contributed to regaining her strength and balance. Over time, she returned to her garden and discovered a renewed zest for life. The exercises became a daily ritual, infusing her days with purpose and joy.

These stories share a common thread: the moment of realization, the turning point when each individual recognized the need for change. For Emma, it was the decision to embrace a structured exercise routine. For David, the shift in perspective came with a reimagined workspace. And for Margaret, rediscovering her passion came from the gentle, yet consistent exercises that became her new routine. These moments of clarity are often accompanied by emotional shifts, as individuals move from frustration and despair to empowerment and hope. They illustrate the emotional impact of recovery, where alleviating back pain translates into increased confidence and renewed enthusiasm for life. No longer constrained by discomfort, these individuals found the freedom to pursue activities that once seemed unreachable.

Through these narratives, a sense of empathy and connection emerges. You may see reflections of your own experiences in their struggles and triumphs. The personal anecdotes and reflections shared here are not just stories; they are invitations to connect, to find inspiration, and to realize that you are not alone on this journey. The path to recovery is paved with the shared wisdom of those who have walked it before, offering guidance and reassurance as you forge your own way forward. As you immerse yourself in these stories, let them serve as reminders of the resilience within you and the possibilities that lie ahead.

Reflection Section: Personal Anecdotes and Insights

- **Exercise**: Reflect on a moment in your life when you faced a similar challenge. What was the turning point that led to change? How can these stories inspire your journey to recovery? Consider journaling your thoughts and insights as a way to deepen your connection to the process and track your progress over time.

8.1 OVERCOMING DOUBT: HOW THEY STAYED COMMITTED

Doubt often creeps in like an uninvited guest, casting shadows over the path to recovery. You might find yourself questioning the effectiveness of exercises, wondering if they can truly make a difference. This skepticism isn't uncommon. Many individuals, at the outset of their recovery, grapple with the same uncertainty. A common refrain echoes: "Can simple exercises really alleviate this pain?" Such doubts are fueled by past experiences—perhaps attempts that fell short, leaving you hesitant to believe in new possibilities. Yet, those who have walked this path before you have shown that doubt can be a catalyst for change, not a barrier. They discovered that, while skepticism might linger, it's the act of trying, of pushing past hesitation, that leads to breakthroughs.

Maintaining commitment in the face of skepticism requires a strategic approach. Start by setting achievable short-term goals. These aren't about instant transformation, but about creating small victories that build confidence. For instance, you might aim to perform a specific stretch daily for a week. These goals act as stepping stones, each one a testament to progress. As you achieve them, they reinforce the belief that change is possible. Another powerful strategy is regularly revisiting your personal motivations. Why did you begin this recovery journey? Perhaps it was the desire to play with your children without pain or to return to a beloved sport. Keeping these motivations at the forefront of your mind can provide a wellspring of strength when doubt threatens to derail your efforts.

A shift in mindset is often the turning point in overcoming doubt. Embracing a growth mindset—where challenges are seen as opportunities for learning rather than insurmountable obstacles—can transform your recovery process. It encourages you to view setbacks not as failures but as valuable lessons. This mindset nurtures patience and persistence, essential qualities when the path seems arduous. It reminds you that progress isn't always linear, but each step, no matter how small, contributes to the larger picture of healing. Cultivating patience allows you to persist through moments of doubt, fostering resilience and adaptability.

For those grappling with doubt, take heart in the stories of others who have triumphed. Consider Tom Kessler, a chronic back pain patient who once believed running was forever out of reach. Despite years of setbacks, Tom's perseverance and the support of his medical team enabled him to overcome his doubts. Through consistent effort and the embrace of new treatments, he alleviated his pain and ran marathons again. His journey illustrates the power of determination and the potential of the human spirit. These stories serve as living proof that doubt can be overcome, and success is attainable with commitment and effort.

As you navigate your own recovery, remember that doubt is natural, but it need not define your journey. With each small victory, you chip away at skepticism, replacing it with confidence and hope. Let the experiences of others inspire you to push through moments of uncertainty, knowing that every effort brings you closer to a life where pain no longer holds sway. Embrace the process with an open heart, and trust in your ability to overcome the challenges ahead.

8.2 BUILDING A SUPPORT NETWORK: THE ROLE OF COMMUNITY

In any endeavor towards healing, the presence of a strong support network can profoundly impact your recovery journey. Imagine the comfort of knowing that you're not alone, that others stand beside you, ready to offer encouragement and practical advice. This kind of support becomes a lifeline, helping you stay motivated and focused on your goals. Emotional support from friends, family, and community members can lift your spirits when challenges arise, offering reassurance and a sense of belonging. Practical support, on the other hand, might involve sharing resources, exchanging tips on effective exercises, or even providing a ride to a physical therapy session. The dual benefits of emotional and practical support create a safety net, ensuring that you have someone to lean on when the going gets tough.

Stories abound of individuals who found strength through their communities. Consider the experience of a busy mother who joined a local support group for individuals dealing with back pain. Within this circle, she not only discovered shared experiences, but also gained valuable insights into managing her condition. The camaraderie and collective wisdom bolstered her resolve, transforming her outlook on recovery. Similarly, a young professional, feeling isolated in his struggles, found solace in online forums dedicated to back health. Engaging in discussions and sharing his progress with others in similar circumstances offered a profound sense of connection and accountability. These community resources became powerful allies, providing encouragement and innovative solutions that might not have emerged in isolation.

The impact of peer encouragement on recovery outcomes is significant. When you share your progress with an accountability partner, you gain a sense of responsibility not only to yourself, but also to someone else invested in your success. This partnership creates a dynamic where progress is celebrated and setbacks are met with understanding and support. The simple act of updating a friend on your achievements or challenges can reinforce your commitment, making the recovery process feel less daunting. This peer support often translates into practical advice, as individuals share what has worked for them and learn from each other's experiences.

Building your own support network may seem daunting, but it begins with small, intentional steps. Reach out to friends and family, sharing your goals and inviting them to be part of your journey. Their encouragement and understanding can be invaluable. Consider engaging in community activities that align with your interests or health goals. Whether it's a local walking club, a yoga class, or a support group meeting, these environments offer opportunities to connect with others who share similar aspirations. The bonds forged in these settings can become sources of inspiration and motivation, reminding you that you're part of a larger community of individuals striving for health and well-being. Each connection strengthens your resolve, creating a tapestry of support that bolsters your efforts and enriches your life.

Interactive Element: Building Your Support Network Action Plan

- **Task**: List three people you can reach out to for support in your recovery. Consider their roles in your life and how they might contribute to your health goals. Identify one community activity or group you can join that aligns with your interests and wellness objectives. Write down the steps you will take to engage with these resources in the coming weeks.

The connections you build and nurture will serve as steadfast companions, guiding you as you navigate the path to recovery and beyond.

8.3 FROM PAIN TO PASSION: HOW RECOVERY CHANGED LIVES

Imagine transforming pain into a source of newfound passion and purpose. For many, overcoming back pain becomes a pivotal moment, opening doors to opportunities previously deemed impossible. Take the story of one individual who, after years of debilitating discomfort, found solace in a fitness routine tailored to their needs. This journey sparked a passion for wellness, leading them to become a fitness advocate. They now inspire others, using their personal experience to guide those facing similar struggles. This shift not only alleviated physical pain but also ignited a sense of purpose, driving them to help others achieve their health goals.

Recovery often acts as a catalyst for change, prompting individuals to explore new career paths. Consider someone who, after successfully managing their back pain, decided to transition into a career in health and wellness. Their firsthand experience fueled a desire to educate others about the importance of maintaining spine health. This career shift not only allowed them to share their knowledge but also provided a sense of fulfillment and satisfaction. The journey from patient to practitioner underscores the transformative power of recovery, highlighting how overcoming adversity can lead to personal and professional growth.

The newfound freedom that comes with recovery can open doors to activities once hindered by pain. Imagine the joy of traveling without limitations, exploring new destinations without the constant worry of discomfort. For those who have endured chronic pain, the ability to pursue hobbies and adventures previously out of reach is truly liberating. Whether it's hiking through a national park or simply gardening in the backyard, these activities become more than just pastimes; they are celebrations of newfound mobility and freedom. The ability to engage in these pursuits enhances quality of life, enriching everyday experiences.

Self-discovery often accompanies the recovery process, leading to greater self-awareness and personal growth. As individuals navigate their path to health, they uncover personal strengths and resilience they never knew they possessed. This journey of self-discovery fosters a sense of empowerment, reminding them of their capacity to overcome challenges. By recognizing and embracing these newfound strengths, individuals are better equipped to tackle future obstacles. This awareness boosts confidence and encourages a proactive approach to health and wellness, paving the way for continued growth and development.

Inspiring others to find their passion as part of their recovery journey is a powerful motivator. Exploring new interests and opportunities can bring joy and fulfillment, transforming the recovery process into a positive and enriching experience. Whether it's taking up a new sport, learning a musical instrument, or volunteering in the community, these activities can foster a sense of purpose and belonging. By encouraging exploration and curiosity, individuals can discover passions that enhance their lives and contribute to their well-being. This mindset shift turns recovery into a journey of self-exploration, leading to a more vibrant and fulfilling life.

8.4 LESSONS LEARNED: ADVICE FROM THOSE WHO'VE BEEN THERE

In the realm of recovery from back pain, practical wisdom from those who have successfully navigated the path, can be invaluable. One of the most emphasized pieces of advice from these individuals is the importance of consistency in routines. Consistency doesn't just mean sticking to a rigid schedule; it means making a habit of the exercises and lifestyle changes that promote healing. Daily routines, no matter how small, lay the foundation for long-term success. Each stretch, each mindful breath, accumulates into something much larger—a healthier, more resilient body. The joy found in small daily improvements is another recurring theme. Recognizing and celebrating these incremental gains, like reduced pain after a walk or increased flexibility from consistent stretching, fuels motivation and reinforces the positive behaviors that lead to recovery.

However, the journey to recovery is not without its pitfalls. Overexertion in the early stages is a common mistake. Eager to reclaim their former strength, many push their bodies too hard, too soon. This can lead to setbacks and prolonged pain. The key is to listen to your body, allowing it to guide your pace. Balancing rest and activity is crucial. Rest is not a sign of weakness but a necessary component of healing. It's important to integrate rest days into your routine, allowing your body the time it needs to repair and rebuild. By alternating between periods of activity and rest, you create a rhythm that sustains your progress without risking injury.

Inspiration often comes from the words of those who have triumphed over adversity. "Progress, not perfection," is a mantra that resonates deeply with many on the path to recovery. It serves as a reminder that the journey is not about achieving an ideal state, but about moving forward, one step at a time. Perfection is an illusion, but progress is tangible and achievable. This mindset encourages patience and self-compassion, allowing individuals to appreciate their journey's unique pace and challenges. Such perspectives can be transformative, shifting the focus from impossible ideals to realistic, meaningful goals.

Reflection and personal growth are integral to the recovery process. Taking the time to reflect on your journey provides valuable insights into what works and what doesn't. Journaling can be a powerful tool in this regard. By documenting your experiences, you create a record of your progress and challenges, which can serve as a roadmap for future endeavors. Self-assessment exercises encourage a more profound understanding of your body's responses and limitations, enabling more informed decisions about your health. These practices foster a sense of ownership and empowerment, as you become an active participant in your recovery.

Reflection Section: Journaling Prompt

- **Prompt**: Reflect on the progress you've made in your recovery journey. What small improvements have you noticed? How have these changes impacted your daily life? Consider writing about a recent challenge you overcame and the lessons you learned from the experience. Use this exercise to acknowledge your achievements and set intentions for continued growth.

As you continue your journey, remember that each lesson learned and each insight gained brings you closer to a life of balance and well-being.

8.5 THE ROAD AHEAD: MAINTAINING YOUR NEW LIFESTYLE

As you tread the path of recovery from back pain, it's crucial to understand that this is not a temporary fix but a long-term commitment to your health. The habits and practices you've cultivated are the foundation of a pain-free life. Continuing these regular exercise routines is vital. They're not just tasks to be ticked off a list; they're your allies in maintaining spine health. Each stretch and strength-building exercise reinforces the stability and flexibility of your back. By integrating these exercises into your daily life, you ensure that your body remains resilient against the stresses of everyday activities. This commitment to movement is a promise to yourself—a pledge to protect the progress you've made.

Equally important is adhering to ergonomic practices. The adjustments you've made to your workspace and daily activities are not mere conveniences; they're essential to your well-being. Proper posture and supportive environments reduce the strain on your spine, preventing the recurrence of pain. Remember that these changes are not static. As your body adapts, so too should your environment. Regularly assess your workspace and lifestyle to ensure they continue to support your health. This might mean adjusting your chair's height or incorporating more breaks during long periods of sitting. These small adjustments play a significant role in maintaining the positive changes you've achieved.

For sustained well-being, setting new, evolving goals is key. These goals keep you engaged and motivated, offering a clear path forward. Start by identifying areas where you can challenge yourself, whether it's increasing the intensity of your workouts or exploring new physical activities. Regularly revisiting and adjusting your plans ensures that they remain relevant and aligned with your capabilities. This dynamic approach prevents stagnation, encouraging continuous improvement and growth. It's about finding the balance between pushing your limits and respecting your body's signals. This balance fosters a sustainable lifestyle that supports both your physical and mental health.

Ongoing monitoring of your progress and health metrics is an invaluable tool in your journey. Using apps and tools designed for health tracking can provide insights into your habits and patterns. These technologies offer a comprehensive view of your progress, highlighting areas of success and those needing attention. By regularly reviewing this data, you can make informed decisions about your routines and adjust them as necessary. This proactive approach empowers you to take charge of your health, ensuring that you remain on track to achieve your goals. It's not just about maintaining the status quo; it's about actively engaging with your health journey.

Finally, embrace the positive changes you have made. Celebrate the milestones in your health and wellness journey, no matter how small they may seem. Each achievement is a testament to your dedication and resilience. Whether it's a day without pain or a new personal best in your fitness routine, take a moment to acknowledge and appreciate these victories. They are the building blocks of a life unburdened by chronic pain. By fully embracing your new lifestyle, you open the door to endless possibilities for growth and fulfillment. Your commitment to maintaining these changes will ensure that your spine health and overall well-being continue to flourish.

CAN YOU HELP?

Let me leave you with a quick reminder. There are hundreds of millions of people across the world suffering from lower back pain, and they're looking for help. If you could spare just a few minutes now to write a short review, you could make a real difference to them.

Simply by sharing your honest opinion of this book and a little about how it's helped you, you'll help new readers find it and gather the information they need to take care of their own back health.

WANT TO HELP OTHERS?

Thank you so much for your support. I wish you good health and happiness as you go forward.

Scan the QR code below.

CONCLUSION

As we come to the end of this journey, I want to take a moment to reflect on the path we've traveled together. Throughout the pages of this book, we've explored the intricacies of lower back pain, uncovering the secrets to relief and long-term recovery. Each chapter has been a stepping stone, guiding you towards a comprehensive understanding of how targeted exercises, lifestyle changes, and a positive mindset can transform your life.

From the anatomy of the spine to the power of proper technique, we've delved into the core principles that underpin a healthy back. You've discovered the importance of tailoring exercises to your unique needs, whether you're an athlete, a senior, or a desk worker. The evidence-based programs outlined in this book provide a roadmap for strengthening your body and alleviating pain, empowering you to take control of your well-being.

But the journey doesn't stop with physical exercises alone. We've explored the profound impact of lifestyle choices on your spine health. Ergonomic adjustments, from your workspace to your daily habits, can make a world of difference in preventing and managing pain. The anti-inflammatory diet and the art of decompression offer natural ways to support your body's healing processes. By integrating these strategies into your daily life, you create a foundation for lasting comfort and mobility.

Perhaps most importantly, we've delved into the mind-body connection, recognizing the power of your thoughts and emotions in shaping your experience of pain. Mindfulness, stress reduction, and the cultivation of resilience are potent tools in your arsenal. By nurturing a positive outlook and embracing the support of others, you create an environment where healing can thrive.

As you close this book, I want you to know that you hold the key to your own well-being. The knowledge and strategies you've gained are yours to implement, adapt, and build upon. Every small change you make, every conscious choice to prioritize your health, is a step towards a life unburdened by back pain. The path may not always be easy, but with consistency and dedication, you have the power to transform your reality.

I encourage you to apply what you've learned, to experiment and find what works best for you. Remember that progress is a journey, not a destination. Celebrate your victories, no matter how small they may seem, and be kind to yourself when challenges arise. You are not alone in this journey. The stories shared within these pages are a testament to the resilience of the human spirit and the possibilities that await when you commit to your well-being.

As you move forward, keep this book as a companion and a guide. Revisit the exercises, the tips, and the insights whenever you need a reminder of your own strength. Share your experiences with others, for in our shared stories, we find comfort and inspiration. Together, we can create a community of support, encouraging one another to live our best lives.

From the bottom of my heart, I want to thank you for trusting me to be a part of your journey. As a retired Sports Chiropractor with over 40 years of experience, I've seen firsthand the transformative power of the strategies outlined in this book. It is my deepest hope that the knowledge and tools you've gained will serve you well, not just in managing back pain, but in embracing a life of vitality and joy.

Remember, your health is your most precious asset. Cherish it, nurture it, and never stop striving for a better tomorrow. The path to a pain-free life is within your reach. With every step you take, you are reclaiming your freedom and writing a new chapter in your story. I believe in you, and I am honored to have been a part of your journey.

Here's to your health, your happiness, and a future filled with endless possibilities. May your spine be strong, your mind be resilient, and your heart be filled with hope. The best is yet to come.

With warmest regards, Dr. K.D. Christensen

REFERENCES

Hopler, Whitney. "Famous Quotes on Service and Well-Being." Center for the Advancement of Well-Being. Accessed February 20, 2025. https://wellbeing.gmu.edu/famous-quotes-on-service-and-well-being/.

"Low Back Pain." June 19, 2023. World Health Organization (WHO). Accessed February 20, 2025. https://www.who.int/news-room/fact-sheets/detail/low-back-pain.

Lumbar Spine: What It Is, Anatomy & Disorders https://my.clevelandclinic.org/health/articles/22396-lumbar-spine

Low Back Pain in Older Adults https://www.spine-health.com/conditions/lower-back-pain/low-back-pain-older-adults

Emerging Challenges and Opportunities in Spine Health https://www.neurologylive.com/view/emerging-challenges-opportunities-spine-health-comprehensive-overview

Acute and chronic low back pain https://pubmed.ncbi.nlm.nih.gov/24994051/

Office ergonomics: Your how-to guide https://www.mayoclinic.org/healthy-lifestyle/adult-health/in-depth/office-ergonomics/art-20046169

Anti-Inflammatory Foods for Optimal Spinal Health https://spinehealth.org/article/anti-inflammatory-foods-for-optimal-spinal-health/

Prevent Back Pain - MyHealthfinder | odphp.health.gov https://odphp.health.gov/myhealthfinder/healthy-living/safety/prevent-back-pain

The Importance of Muscle Hydration https://www.athletico.com/2021/08/23/the-importance-of-muscle-hydration/

Exercise therapy for chronic low back pain - PMC https://pmc.ncbi.nlm.nih.gov/articles/PMC8477273/

Posture and back health https://www.health.harvard.edu/pain/posture-and-back-health

The Health Benefits of Tai Chi for Seniors | Aegis Living https://www.aegisliving.com/resource-center/the-health-benefits-of-tai-chi-for-seniors/

Office ergonomics: Your how-to guide https://www.mayoclinic.org/healthy-lifestyle/adult-health/in-depth/office-ergonomics/art-20046169

Find the Best Back Pain App for You https://www.healthcentral.com/condition/back-pain/best-back-pain-apps

Spine-health: Trusted Information on Back Pain and Neck Pain https://www.spine-health.com/

3D posture analysis - Physiolistic https://www.physiolistic.co.uk/3dpostureanalysis

14 Emerging Wearable Health Technologies Transforming ... https://www.forbes.com/councils/forbestechcouncil/2024/06/11/14-emerging-wearable-health-technologies-transforming-remote-care/

Creating a SMART Plan of Care for Physical Therapy https://www.clinicient.com/blog/creating-a-smart-plan-of-care-for-physical-therapy/

Recover Athletics on the App Store https://apps.apple.com/us/app/recover-athletics/id1488347465

How to Overcome Plateaus in the Rehabilitation Process https://www.goldstarrehab.com/parent-resources/how-to-overcome-plateaus-in-the-rehabilitation-process

Chiropractic Treatments for Lower Back Pain - Spine-health https://www.spine-health.com/treatment/chiropractic/chiropractic-treatments-lower-back-pain

The interaction between stress and chronic pain through ... https://www.sciencedirect.com/science/article/abs/pii/S0149763419305792

Mindfulness meditation–based pain relief: a mechanistic ... https://pmc.ncbi.nlm.nih.gov/articles/PMC4941786/

Cognitive-behavioral therapy for patients with chronic pain https://pmc.ncbi.nlm.nih.gov/articles/PMC5999451/

The 10 Best Yoga Poses for Back Pain https://www.healthline.com/health/fitness-exercise/yoga-for-back-pain

How to avoid exercise injuries - MedlinePlus https://medlineplus.gov/ency/patientinstructions/000859.htm

Dynamic Warmups for Athletes: Exercises for Performance ... https://blog.nasm.org/dynamic-warm-ups-for-athletes-injury-prevention-and-sports-performance-benefits

The Benefits of Cross Training for Your Back https://magmafitness.ca/blogs/magma-blog/the-benefits-of-cross-training-for-your-back?srsltid=AfmBOordeBXw47JuP_Wg1w0ReOM-fTH9N6ID6Qbt3jC3vyj391Tv639u

Proprioception Exercises for Better Balance and Body ... https://www.healthline.com/health/fitness/proprioception-exercises

From Back Pain to Back in Action https://www.medstarhealth.org/news-and-publications/patient-stories-and-testimonials/from-back-pain-to-back-in-action

Psychological therapies for the management of chronic pain https://pmc.ncbi.nlm.nih.gov/articles/PMC3986332/

Community support for injured patients: A scoping review ... https://pmc.ncbi.nlm.nih.gov/articles/PMC10833531/

Tom Ressler: Chronic Back Pain Patient Story https://my.clevelandclinic.org/patient-stories/557-caregiver-runs-marathon-after-enduring-debilitating-chronic-pain

Made in the USA
Monee, IL
19 October 2026

66036212R00079